T0226958

Perioperative Considerations in the Surgical Patient

Editor

JEFFREY E. SHOOK

CLINICS IN PODIATRIC MEDICINE AND SURGERY

www.podiatric.theclinics.com

Consulting Editor
THOMAS J. CHANG

January 2019 • Volume 36 • Number 1

ELSEVIER

1600 John F. Kennedy Boulevard ● Suite 1800 ● Philadelphia, Pennsylvania, 19103-2899

http://www.theclinics.com

CLINICS IN PODIATRIC MEDICINE AND SURGERY Volume 36, Number 1
January 2019 ISSN 0891-8422, ISBN-13: 978-0-323-65489-0

Editor: Lauren Boyle
Developmental Editor: Sara Watkins

Clinics in Podiatric Medicine and Surgery (ISSN 0891-8422) is published quarterly by Elsevier Inc., 360 Park Avenue South, New York, NY 10010-1710. Months of issue are January, April, July, and October. Business and Editorial Offices: 1600 John F. Kennedy Blvd., Ste. 1800, Philadelphia, PA 19103-2899. Customer Service Office: 3251 Riverport Lane, Maryland Heights, MO 63043. Periodicals postage paid at New York, NY and additional mailing offices. Subscription prices are $304.00 per year for US individuals, $574.00 per year for US institutions, $100.00 per year for US students and residents, $382.00 per year for Canadian individuals, $693.00 for Canadian institutions, $439.00 for international individuals, $693.00 per year for international institutions and $220.00 per year for Canadian and foreign students/residents. To receive student/resident rate, orders must be accompanied by name of affiliated institution, date of term, and the *signature* of program/residency coordinator on institution letterhead. Orders will be billed at individual rate until proof of status is received. Foreign air speed delivery is included in all *Clinics* subscription prices. All prices are subject to change without notice. POSTMASTER: Send address changes to *Clinics in Podiatric Medicine and Surgery*, Elsevier Health Sciences Division, Subscription Customer Service, 3251 Riverport Lane, Maryland Heights, MO 63043. **Customer Service: 1-800-654-2452 (US). From outside of the US, call 314-447-8871. Fax: 314-447-8029. E-mail: JournalsCustomerService-usa@elsevier.com (for print support); JournalsOnlineSupport-usa@elsevier. com (for online support).**

Reprints. For copies of 100 or more of articles in this publication, please contact the Commercial Reprints Department, Elsevier Inc., 360 Park Avenue South, New York, NY 10010-1710. Tel.: 212-633-3874; Fax: 212-633-3820; E-mail: reprints@elsevier.com.

Clinics in Podiatric Medicine and Surgery is covered in *MEDLINE/PubMed (Index Medicus)* and *EMBASE/Excerpta Medica.*

Contributors

CONSULTING EDITOR

THOMAS J. CHANG, DPM
Clinical Professor and Past Chairman, Department of Podiatric Surgery, California College of Podiatric Medicine, Faculty, The Podiatry Institute, Redwood Orthopedic Surgery Associates, Santa Rosa, California

EDITOR

JEFFREY E. SHOOK, DPM
Satilla Foot and Ankle, Waycross, Georgia; Adjunct Faculty, St. Vincent Charity Medical Center, Cleveland, Ohio; Adjunct Faculty, Kent State University College of Podiatric Medicine, Independence, Ohio

AUTHORS

MIAN BILAL ALAM, MD
Fellow, Department of Adult Cardiovascular Medicine, Joan C. Edwards School of Medicine, Marshall University, Huntington, West Virginia

AMANDA BENSON, MD
Staff, General Anesthesiology and Critical Care, Assistant Clinical Professor of Anesthesiology, Cleveland Clinic Lerner College of Medicine, Cleveland Clinic, Cleveland, Ohio

BRADLEY BENSON, DPM
Podiatric Medicine and Surgery Residency Program, Resident PGYIII, St. Vincent Charity Medical Center, Cleveland, Ohio

JOHN BORZOK, DPM
Second Year Resident, Podiatric Medicine and Surgery Residency Program, University Hospital, Newark, New Jersey

JOHN BOYD, DPM
Third Year Resident, Section of Podiatry, Department of Surgery, St. Vincent Charity Medical Center, Cleveland, Ohio

DANIEL BULLARD, DPM
PGY II, Second Year Resident, St. Vincent Charity Medical Center, Cleveland, Ohio

DYLAN M. CARLISLE, DPM
Third Year Resident, DeKalb Medical Center, Decatur, Georgia

PRESTON CARR, MS
Medical Student, Kent State University College of Podiatric Medicine, Independence, Ohio

RICHARD CHMIELEWSKI, MD
Director, Infectious Control, Section of Podiatry, Department of Surgery, St. Vincent Charity Medical Center, Cleveland, Ohio

KEITH D. COOK, DPM, FACFAS
Director, Podiatric Medical Education, Assistant Director, Podiatry Department, University Hospital, Newark, New Jersey

ALEX DAWOODIAN, DPM
Resident PGYIII, Podiatric Medicine and Surgery Residency Program, St. Vincent Charity Medical Center, Cleveland, Ohio

DUANE J. EHREDT Jr, DPM, FACFAS
Assistant Professor, Division of Foot and Ankle Surgery, Kent State University College of Podiatric Medicine, Independence, Ohio; Surgical Faculty, Podiatric Medicine and Surgery Residency Program, St. Vincent Charity Medical Center, Cleveland, Ohio

AHMAD ETER, MD
Hospitalist, Nephrologist, Princeton Community Hospital, Princeton, West Virginia

JARED L. MOON, DPM, FACFAS
Attending Staff, St. Mary Medical Center, Hobart, Indiana

KAREN M. MOON, DPM
Third Year Resident, DeKalb Medical Center, Decatur, Georgia

DOUGLAS J. OPLER, MD
Assistant Professor, Department of Psychiatry, Rutgers New Jersey Medical School, Newark, New Jersey

PARIS PAYTON, DPM
Department of Podiatric Surgery, St. Vincent Charity Medical Center, Cleveland, Ohio

DOUG RICHIE, DPM
Private Practice, Alamitos-Seal Beach Podiatry Group, Seal Beach, California; Clinical Associate Professor, Department of Biomechanics, California School of Podiatric Medicine at Samuel Merritt University, Oakland, California; Clinical Associate Professor of Podiatric Medicine and Surgery, Western University of Health Sciences, Pomona, California

RAMEEZ SAYYED, MD, FACC, FSCAI
Associate Professor, Department of Adult Cardiovascular Medicine, Joan C. Edwards School of Medicine, Marshall University, Huntington, West Virginia

JEFFREY E. SHOOK, DPM
Satilla Foot and Ankle, Waycross, Georgia; Adjunct Faculty, St. Vincent Charity Medical Center, Cleveland, Ohio; Adjunct Faculty, Kent State University College of Podiatric Medicine, Independence, Ohio

FADWA SUMREIN, DO
Endocrinology Fellow, Department of Medicine, Rutgers New Jersey Medical School, Newark, New Jersey

H. JOHN VISSER, DPM, FACFAS
Director, Foot and Ankle Surgery Residency, SSM Health DePaul Hospital, St Louis, Missouri

JESSE WOLFE, DPM
Resident, Foot and Ankle Surgery Residency, SSM Health DePaul Hospital, St Louis, Missouri

JOSHUA WOLFE, DPM, MHA
Resident, Foot and Ankle Surgery Residency, SSM Health DePaul Hospital, St Louis, Missouri

Contents

There are multiple challenges the podiatric surgeon faces while attempting to treat patients in the perioperative setting. Given the aging and increasingly complex surgical population, preoperative evaluation is of utmost importance to mitigate unnecessary risks and to optimize patient outcomes. This article reviews key preoperative considerations, patient evaluation, and factors affecting selection of anesthetic technique.

Although rare, deep vein thrombosis (DVT) and pulmonary embolism remain a concern for foot and ankle surgeons. Most prophylactic measures against DVT formation are synthesized from orthopedic hip and knee data, and therefore the routine use of these recommendations may place patients at risk for complications associated with unnecessary prophylaxis. In this article we review and present the most current literature specific to venous thromboembolism (VTE) in foot and ankle surgery. It is clear that, given our current literature, a case-by-case approach for VTE prophylaxis should be used following foot and ankle surgery.

The literature for prevention of surgical infection related primarily to foot and ankle surgery is sparse, with most attention on total joint replacement and abdominal surgery. Attention should be paid to preoperative, intraoperative, and postoperative elements, which can have an effect on the development of postoperative infection. Although antibiotic prophylaxis typically is discussed in isolation, inclusion of this step into the process enhances the overall evaluation of surgery with respect to infection. This evolution provides for better patient outcomes and decreases the likelihood of an infection incurred after foot and ankle surgery.

> Treating patients with kidney disease can be both a difficult and a complex process. Understanding how to care for patients who have kidney disease is essential for lowering perioperative as well as periprocedural morbidity and mortality. The primary aim in renal evaluation and care is to control and mitigate factors that may result in acute kidney injury (AKI) and/or cause further decline in renal function. It is essential for the foot and ankle specialist to recognize patients who are predisposed to developing or already have impairment of renal function.

> Diabetes mellitus is a devastating disease that has reached epidemic proportions. The surgical patient with diabetes is at increased risk for developing complications when compared with patients without diabetes. A comprehensive preoperative work-up must be performed, including ancillary studies, with optimization of the patient's glucose levels during the perioperative period to decrease the chance of developing surgical complications. A multispecialty team approach for the care of patients with diabetes should be used to produce successful surgical outcomes.

> The ability to identify and guide evaluation of the patient with cardiac disease represents a necessary skill for success in surgery of the foot and ankle. Common risk factors, such as diabetes and peripheral arterial disease, are encountered in podiatric practice. Recognition of patients at risk for cardiac disease and a predilection for sustaining a major adverse cardiac event perioperatively advocates for preoperative cardiology consultation. Identification of risk factors, assessment of functional capacity, and appropriate work-up mitigate any untoward cardiac events surrounding surgery. This optimization results from appropriate medical and interventional treatment plans directed at minimizing or eliminating identified risks factors.

> Rheumatoid arthritis is a complex disease state with multiple associated comorbidities. Perioperative evaluation of the rheumatoid patient from a multidisciplinary approach is necessary to achieve favorable outcomes. A complete history and physical, laboratory, cervical, cardiovascular, pulmonary, and medication assessment before surgery should be performed. Educating the patient on potential complications, such as wound dehiscence, infection, and venous thromboembolism, as well as general postoperative expectations, is essential when evaluating the rheumatoid patient for surgery.

> Surgical treatment of the elderly can be a very difficult and complex endeavor. Appropriate and thorough evaluation of this group of patients is essential to identify surgical candidates who may be at increased risk for developing age-related problems, such as cognitive impairment or postoperative delirium. Involvement of family members and ancillary caregivers is ideal. In order to optimize surgical results, communication of goals of surgery and expectations of patients in order to achieve these goals is paramount. Physical therapy assessment of the elderly will give input on patients' capacity to perform needed changes in ambulatory status after surgery.

> Obese patients are at higher risk for surgical complications and consist of a large portion of podiatric patients. Obese patients are additionally at increased risk of developing specific podiatric conditions, and it is important to be able to identify and appropriately treat these conditions accordingly. Initially, conservative treatment is adequate for a variety of pathologic conditions related to obesity. Occasionally surgical intervention is warranted depending on the severity and lack of response to conservative measures. Arthrodesis-type procedures are often preferable and may be necessary, as opposed to periarticular osteotomy, in obese patients even if the deformity is flexible.

> Foot and ankle surgery can impose significant hardship on a patient when carrying out their essential activities of daily living including mobility, sourcing and preparing food, as well as maintaining personal hygiene. Pre-operative planning between the surgeon, patient and caregivers can circumvent most of the challenges imposed by the post-operative restrictions of foot and ankle surgery. Depending on the weight bearing status of the operated extremity, a wide array of durable medical equipment devices are available to provide mobility and safety for the patient. Various devices are also available to protect the patient and the operative site during bathing. Pre-operative gait training can be valuable in selecting the most appropriate mobility aid for the patient, assuring safe ambulation while keeping the operated extremity protected.

CLINICS IN PODIATRIC MEDICINE AND SURGERY

THE CLINICS ARE AVAILABLE ONLINE!
Access your subscription at:
www.theclinics.com

Foreword

Perioperative Considerations in the Surgical Patient

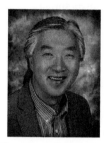

Thomas J. Chang, DPM
Consulting Editor

Although this publication is titled *Clinics in Podiatric Medicine and Surgery*, I will admit that the prior issues have been slanted a bit in the surgical direction. Over the past months, I felt an obligation to balance this out by dedicating an issue to a focus on medicine. On the top of my list is the perioperative management of our surgical patients. Dr Shook shared this vision, and so this issue was born. Our students currently sit alongside allopathic medical students in most of their basic science courses and train directly with allopathic residents in medical and surgical residencies. As we move toward parity with our allopathic colleagues in all aspects of professional life, there is an expectation and sense of responsibility to be more aware and involved with the medical comanagement of our patients. This long overdue topic area will serve as an up-to-date review for some and an important initiation for others.

I applaud Dr Shook's foresight in identifying these pertinent specialty areas we encounter in our surgical practices. He has brought together known experts in these specific areas, and I am grateful for their time and efforts. I am hopeful these articles will provide some inspiration for further exploration and research, and more importantly, will assist us all in more complete and successful management of our surgical population.

Thomas J. Chang, DPM
Redwood Orthopedic Surgery Associates
208 Concourse Boulevard
Santa Rosa, CA 95403, USA

E-mail address:
thomaschang14@comcast.net

Clin Podiatr Med Surg 36 (2019) xi
https://doi.org/10.1016/j.cpm.2018.09.004
0891-8422/19/© 2018 Published by Elsevier Inc.

podiatric.theclinics.com

Preface

Perioperative Considerations in the Surgical Patient

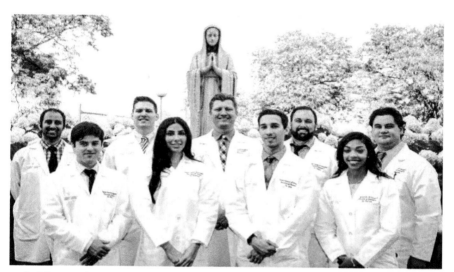

St. Vincent Charity Medical Center Podiatric Surgical Residency Program, 2017-2018

This issue of *Clinics in Podiatric Medicine and Surgery*, devoted to "Perioperative Considerations in the Surgical Patient," is designed to update the foot and ankle surgeon on prevalent medical problems, which affect the conditions and process surrounding any given patient's surgery. The main focus is to emphasize the importance of surgeons approaching a surgical candidate as a physician, and not simply as a technician completing a task. Not only should the surgery be tailored to each patient, but the perioperative approach should also be individualized to each patient's needs and medical requirements in order to obtain the best possible surgical result.

I would like to thank all of the authors who contributed to this issue. I appreciate your expertise reflected in these articles and the time spent on the content of this issue. Special acknowledgment is extended to the 2017/2018 residency program at St Vincent Charity Medical Center, Cleveland, Ohio. It is difficult enough to actively participate in a demanding residency program; I appreciate the extra commitment that was made to contribute to this project.

This issue would not have been possible without the never-ending assistance and editing from Donna Perzeski. Donna has supported the education of future podiatrists for decades and serves as the librarian at the Ohio College of Podiatric Medicine. She has been the heart and soul of this institution for the past 38 years. I would also like to personally thank two podiatrists. First, to my mentor: Gerard V. Yu, DPM: "Give a man

Clin Podiatr Med Surg 36 (2019) xiii–xiv
https://doi.org/10.1016/j.cpm.2018.09.003
0891-8422/19/© 2018 Published by Elsevier Inc.

podiatric.theclinics.com

a fish and feed him for a day, teach a man how to fish and feed him for a lifetime." Thanks for teaching me how to fish. We miss you! Second, to my friend: Larry Osher, DPM: thanks for pulling me up during the bad times and giving me balance during the good times. Simply put, you are the best person I know and the epitome of a friend, thank you. I would also like to thank my wife, Jessi, and our four children, Sebastian, Aryel, Evan, and Liam, for their support and patience.

Jeffrey E. Shook, DPM
Satilla Foot and Ankle
545 Knight Avenue
Waycross, GA 31501, USA

Adjunct Faculty
St. Vincent Charity Medical Center
Cleveland, OH 44115, USA

Adjunct Faculty
Kent State University College of Podiatric Medicine
Independence, OH 44131, USA

E-mail address:
Jshook7@kent.edu

Preoperative Anesthetic Considerations in the Podiatric Surgical Candidate

Bradley Benson, DPM[a],*, Amanda Benson, MD[b]

KEYWORDS

- Preoperative evaluation • Anesthesia • Podiatry • Lower extremity • Diabetic

KEY POINTS

- History and physical examination are key to guiding appropriate preoperative workup.
- Given the comorbidities often present in the podiatric patient, preoperative evaluation and optimization should have a special focus on cardiovascular, pulmonary, endocrine, and renal systems.
- There a several anesthetic options, including general anesthesia, monitored anesthesia care, and neuraxial and regional anesthesia, each with their unique advantages and disadvantages to consider in podiatric surgery.

INTRODUCTION

There can be significant confusion surrounding the needs of the anesthesia team when considering operative management of the podiatric patient. The goal of both the surgeon and the anesthesiologist should always be to minimize perioperative patient risk. This is best achieved by thorough preoperative assessment, individualized evaluation of comorbid diseases, and optimization of these conditions. With an understanding of the anesthetic needs and risks based on the procedural and patient factors, an efficient evaluation can be performed that suits the needs of the surgeon, as well as the anesthesiologist, and limits surgical delays and cancellations. Although this review provides a basic approach for preoperative workup, it is the responsibility of the surgeon, as well as the anesthesiologist, to maintain an open line of communication with mutual respect to provide the best perioperative care.

Disclosures: None.
[a] Podiatric Medicine and Surgery Residency Program, Saint Vincent Charity Medical Center, 2351 East 22nd Street, Cleveland, OH 44115, USA; [b] General Anesthesiology and Critical Care, Cleveland Clinic Lerner College of Medicine, Cleveland Clinic, 9500 Euclid Avenue, Cleveland, OH 44195, USA
* Corresponding author.
E-mail address: bradleybenson13@gmail.com

Clin Podiatr Med Surg 36 (2019) 1–19
https://doi.org/10.1016/j.cpm.2018.08.001
0891-8422/19/© 2018 Elsevier Inc. All rights reserved.
podiatric.theclinics.com

PREANESTHETIC EVALUATION

When considering a preoperative workup, one must consider the definition a preanesthetic evaluation. Per the American Society of Anesthesiologists (ASA): *Preanesthesia evaluation consists of the consideration of information from multiple sources that may include that patient's medical records, interview, physical examination, and findings from medical tests and evaluations.* Starting with medical records, interview and physical examination will help to determine the need for additional testing or consultations. Although it may seem obvious, a diligent examination is necessary to confirm the legitimacy of current medical records but also to evaluate for undiagnosed disease processes, which may affect the perioperative care. For instance, increased lower extremity swelling or coarse breath sounds may be indicative of decompensated heart failure and a harsh systolic murmur may prompt a preoperative workup for aortic stenosis.

It can be beneficial to preemptively order basic laboratory tests and tests such as an electrocardiogram (ECG) or chest radiograph, as this can expedite time to operation for elective procedures and help avoid cancellation in certain instances. The ASA provides some guidelines for preoperative testing. Many institutions (hospitals and surgery centers) have preoperative testing requirements based strictly on medical history. In general, it is recommended to consider surgical patients on a case by case situation to obtain necessary preoperative information, but also to streamline the process at the same time. This again highlights the importance of establishing a good relationship and open communication among the surgeon, anesthesiologist, and the primary care physician. This dialogue will ensure discussion of important factors, such as patient's functional status, invasiveness of procedure, type of anesthesia required for performance of procedure, and, most importantly, clear understanding of patient's cardiac, pulmonary, and renal history.

The ASA Physical Status Classification System allows a fast and easy stratification of the patient's overall health status. Ranging from an ASA score of 1 to 6, the scale represents the severity of comorbid disease present preoperatively, in addition to whether the procedure is emergent.[1,2] A description of each score and examples are provided in **Table 1**. It should be emphasized that the ASA classification does not infer operative risk. Just as important is the known inadequacy of interobserver agreement using this system, especially when a nonanesthesia-trained health care provider is involved. This has become increasingly important in today's medical world of "fast track," outpatient surgery in which facilities such as surgery centers will take care of only ASA 1 or ASA 2 patients. Accuracy of initial ASA classification by the treating surgeon becomes very important in this scenario. Hurwitz and colleagues[1] recommended review of ASA classification with the supplementation of examples as to appropriate classification of a given patient based on disease burden or physical status (refer to **Table 2**). In this study, after examples were reviewed, the difference in accuracy between anesthesia-trained and nonanesthesia-trained heath care providers was statistically insignificant, and, in fact, the nonanesthesia-trained providers were slightly more accurate.[1] It should be emphasized that the ASA classification primarily exists as a means of communication between health care professionals with regards to a given patient's physical status. Sometimes patients with significant comorbidities and higher ASA status may require postponement of a procedure to medically optimize the patient before surgery and minimize the attendant risks of the surgery and anesthesia.

This particular classification system, although the most widely used, does not account for unique factors specific to a given surgical procedure. This is an important

Table 1
American Society of Anesthesiologists (ASA) physical classification system

ASA Physical Status Class	Definition	Examples, Including, but Not Limited to
I	A healthy patient	Healthy, nonsmoking, no or minimal alcohol use
II	A patient with mild systemic disease	Mild diseases only without substantive functional limitations. Examples include (but not limited to) current smoker, social alcohol drinker, pregnancy, obesity (30< BMI <40), well-controlled DM/HTN, mild lung disease
III	A patient with severe systemic disease	Substantive functional limitations; one or more moderate to severe diseases. Examples include (but not limited to) poorly controlled DM or HTN, COPD, morbid obesity (BMI >40), active hepatitis, alcohol dependence or abuse, implanted pacemaker, moderate reduction of ejection fraction, ESRD undergoing regularly scheduled dialysis, premature infant PCA <60 wk, history (>3 mo) of MI, CVA, TIA, or CAD/stents
IV	A patient with severe systemic disease that is a constant threat to life	Examples include (but not limited to) recent (<3 mo) MI, CVA, TIA, or CAD/stents, ongoing cardiac ischemia or severe valve dysfunction, severe reduction of ejection fraction, sepsis, DIC, ARDS, or ESRD not undergoing regularly scheduled dialysis
V	A moribund patient who is not expected to survive without the operation	Examples include (but not limited to) ruptured abdominal/thoracic aneurysm, massive trauma, intracranial bleed with mass effect, ischemic bowel in the face of significant cardiac pathology or multiple organ/system dysfunction
VI	A declared brain-dead patient whose organs are being removed for donor purposes	

The addition of "E" denoted emergency surgery: an emergency is defined as existing when delay in treatment of the patient would lead to a significant increase in the threat to life or body part.

Abbreviations: ARDS, acute respiratory distress syndrome; BMI, body mass index; CAD, coronary artery disease; COPD, chronic obstructive pulmonary disease; CVA, cerebrovascular accident; DIC, disseminated intravascular coagulation; DM, diabetes mellitus; ESRD, end-stage renal disease; HTN, hypertension; MI, myocardial infarction; PCA, post conceptual age; TIA, transient ischemic attack.

Adapted from American Society of Anesthesiologists. ASA Physical Status Classification System. Available at: asahq.org/resources/clinical-information/asa-physical-status-classification-system. Accessed May 22, 2018; with permission.

Table 2
Correct ASA physical status classification for each case and comorbidities from ASA-approved examples

Case No.	ASA Physical Status Class	Patient's Comorbidities from ASA-Approved Examples
1	III	BMI >40
2	II	Controlled HTN, current smoker
3	III	Poorly controlled DM, controlled HTN
4	II	Mild lung disease (controlled asthma, mild OSA), obesity (30< BMI <40)
5	II	Mild lung disease (controlled asthma), controlled DM
6	II	Current smoker, alcohol use
7	III	Controlled HTN, ESRD undergoing regularly scheduled dialysis
8	III	Obesity (30< BMI <40), controlled HTN, history of MI, COPD, poorly controlled DM, ESRD undergoing regularly scheduled dialysis
9	II	Obesity (30< BMI <40), controlled HTN
10	I	Healthy 81 y old

Abbreviations: ASA, American Society of Anesthesiologists; BMI, body mass index; COPD, chronic obstructive pulmonary disease; DM, diabetes mellitus; ESRD, end-stage renal disease; HTN, hypertension; MI, myocardial infarction; OSA, obstructive sleep apnea.

Adapted from American Society of Anesthesiologists. ASA Physical Status Classification System. Available at: asahq.org/resources/clinical-information/asa-physical-status-classification-system. Accessed May 22, 2018; with permission.

limitation. Multiple attempts have been made to address this shortcoming; however, they have fallen short. When considering overall perioperative risk, the surgical risk is often greater than the anesthetic risk. However, with the advent of minimally invasive and microsurgical techniques, this trend may be changing. Age older than 85 years, significant comorbidity, and type of procedure were the strongest predictors of adverse events according to Fleisher and colleagues[3] when considering the 65 and older cohort.

PREOPERATIVE MEDICAL HISTORY

As mentioned previously, there is no replacement for a thorough medical history and physical examination when assessing a patient preoperatively. The goal is to elucidate the current medical conditions, known and previously unknown, and determine the relative stability of these conditions. This helps to direct whether further testing is warranted or additional time is needed to medically optimize the patient. An understanding of the type of operation, as well as any pathologic etiology that has led to the patient's current state is necessary as well. Knowledge of treatments attempted in the past will also paint a clearer picture of the patient's overall status.

Questions surrounding past medical history, past surgeries, allergies, current medications, and drug and alcohol use are all well documented as necessary portions to a thorough evaluation. In addition, emphasis should be placed on a comprehensive review of systems to shed light on undiagnosed disease processes. By the nature of the patients who podiatrists treat, they are attuned to those with peripheral vascular disease possibly more than any other providers. Simply asking questions with regard to difficulty with walking at certain distances can reveal symptoms of claudication. The correlation between peripheral vascular disease and coronary artery disease cannot be understated. Revealing these symptoms before surgery and pursuing additional workup has the potential to substantially reduce perioperative anesthetic and surgical risk.

The need for vascular workup in the podiatric patient is well-known; however, equally important and sometimes overlooked are risk factors for severe reflux and sleep apnea. These are readily identifiable, such as sleeping with the head elevated, snoring, daytime somnolence, hypertension, or obesity. A high suspicion for these conditions should prompt further evaluation, or at a minimum strict preoperative precautions for aspiration risk and perioperative monitoring with pulse oximetry.

PHYSICAL EXAMINATION

In addition to the history, a detailed physical examination is essential to the preoperative evaluation. Weight and body mass index (BMI) are important reflections of the patient's physical health and risk for multiple comorbidities, and are essential for proper dosing of medications perioperatively. Establishing baseline vitals, including heart rate, blood pressure, oxygen saturation on room air, temperature, and respiratory rate can give insight into the medical stability of conditions such as hypertension, pulmonary disease, and arrhythmias, such as atrial fibrillation. It also gives a benchmark for perioperative monitoring, as patients should be kept as close to their baseline vitals as possible to minimize cardiac, pulmonary, renal, and cerebrovascular morbidity.

Auscultation can provide important insights about cardiopulmonary health. Care should be taken to listen for heart murmurs, rubs, or arrhythmias, as well as abnormal lung sounds, such as wheezes, rhonchi, or rales. Examination also should look for signs of heart failure, including jugular venous distention, ascites, hepatomegaly, and peripheral edema, as well as indicators of significant underlying lung disease, including clubbing of digits, accessory muscle use, baseline oxygen requirement, and perioral cyanosis. As mentioned before, of significant importance to the podiatric surgeon is the evaluation and documentation of peripheral perfusion via palpable pulses, noninvasive vascular studies (ankle-brachial index/pulse volume recording) or advanced diagnostic procedures as needed.

Any abnormalities on physical examination should be met with further questions, appropriate consultation to specialists if indicated, and possibly further testing, such as cardiac stress testing or pulmonary function tests. Previously literature has suggested that if a patient has the capacity to walk 1 to 2 flights of stairs with minimal physical duress, they can likely endure the physical demands of anesthesia without further workup to the cardiovascular or respiratory systems.[4] Current evidence and guidelines support this assertion for most low-risk and intermediate-risk procedures. Cardiac and pulmonary workup is not recommended unless there is evidence of a decompensated condition on history or physical examination. In most instances, the primary care physician will have a better working knowledge of the patient's baseline medical status and, ultimately, the best understanding of whether or not a particular patient is medically optimized for surgery. At present, most patients undergo far more preoperative testing than is necessary, which underscores the necessity for good communication among the surgeon, primary care physician, and anesthesiologist well in advance of the day of surgery.

Perhaps of more importance to the anesthesia team is the airway examination., Nonetheless, it is still important for surgeons to understand the basic predictors of a difficult airway. Physical characteristics of difficult intubation by conventional means of direct laryngoscopy include Mallampati score (distance from base of tongue to roof of mouth), size of mouth opening, tongue size, mobility of the cervical spine and jaw, thyromental distance, and interincisor distance. Surgeons should ask if the patient has ever had difficulty with anesthesia. In these instances, the anesthesiologist usually informs the patient of difficulty with intubation for any potential surgeries in the future. Also, if difficulty to intubate or difficulty with anesthesia has been ascertained during surgical preoperative evaluation, anesthesia records should be obtained and made available for the anesthesia team before surgery. Even more important than ease of intubation, is predicting ease of mask ventilation. Factors such as a large face and neck circumference, limited jaw protrusion, lack of teeth, and excess facial hair are all associated with difficult mask ventilation. When multiple predictors are present, anesthesiologists may elect to use nontraditional tools or in some cases, to pursue an awake intubation for patient safety. Dental health can also be important to note, as poor dentition can lead to accidental tooth dislodgement and puts the patient at risk for infection. This is particularly significant when surgical implants are planned.

Obstructive sleep apnea (OSA) is present in a large proportion of the population and can often go undiagnosed. Risk factors include obesity, hypertension, snoring, older age, larger waist to hip ratio, male sex, daytime drowsiness, and large neck circumference (>17″ in adult men and >16″ in adult women).[5,6] Patients with several of these risk factors should be sent for polysomnogram and monitored closely with pulse oximetry in the perioperative setting. A common preoperative screening tool for OSA is the STOP-Bang questionnaire. STOP-BANG is an acronym that stands for Snoring, Tired, Observed apnea, Hypertension, BMI, Age, Neck circumference, and Gender. The first 4 elements are simple yes and no questions that are combined with the last 4 objective findings to give a screening for OSA.[5]

Some of the previously mentioned items, such as the Mallampati score, are not germane to the surgeon's knowledge base or typical history-taking practices. Nevertheless, many of the items mentioned in the airway section should be added to the preoperative evaluation. The surgeon should be cognizant of these issues, as they will certainly affect the anesthesia plan for a proposed surgery. As an example, if you have a 55-year-old man who needs to have a simple digital arthroplasty under monitored anesthesia care (MAC)/local anesthesia but has a history of sleep apnea, an 18-inch collar size, and a full beard, what is the appropriate course of action? This patient example is not uncommon and poses multiple issues with respect to airway management for the anesthesiologist. This is an instance in which the anesthesia team needs to be notified well in advance of the surgery and potentially have a formal preoperative evaluation done to avoid any delay on the day of surgery while still providing the safest anesthesia technique to complete the surgery.

Finally, it is important to evaluate and document any neurologic issues that may present during the preoperative examination. This includes cranial nerves, gait, muscle strength, deep tendon reflexes, sensory evaluation, speech, and mental status. It is critical to document deficits from prior strokes, neuropathy, or other neurologic diseases or injuries before surgery to help determine whether postoperative changes are present. In addition, patients with waxing and waning diseases, such as multiple sclerosis, should be asked about triggers and most recent flare ups.

COMORBIDITIES AND ANESTHESIA

The surgical population is becoming older and more ill. The preoperative history and examination already discussed help to identify comorbid conditions that may complicate the perioperative period. Involvement of the proper consultants is essential to help manage issues stemming from these comorbidities. However, as a leader of the surgical team, a basic understanding of the perioperative considerations of some commonly encountered conditions is important and reviewed here.

Pulmonary

Pulmonary health is of great importance when considering an anesthetic plan. The history and physical examination should provide insight into the patient's pulmonary function and help to identify any issues, diagnosed or otherwise. Unrecognized lung disease can manifest as inability to exercise, dyspnea, or chronic cough. Decreased breath sounds, rhonchi, wheezes, or prolonged expiratory phase are often associated with obstructive lung disease.[7] Restrictive lung disease typically manifests with dyspnea and desaturations. Pulmonary function tests, arterial blood gas, and exercise testing are almost never indicated before lower extremity surgery. However, many patients with chronic lung disease have undergone these tests in the past and reviewing such records can provide additional information regarding the severity of their pulmonary impairment.[8–10] Chest radiograph also can be helpful and is reasonable when considering preoperative workup, but should not be routinely obtained. In a meta-analysis of 14,390 surgical patients who received a chest radiograph preoperatively, 140 had unexpected abnormalities, and only 14 actually changed perioperative management.[11] Although there is a correlation between advanced age and more abnormal findings on chest radiograph,[12] the recommendations remain that preoperative chest radiograph is reserved for those with severe pulmonary disease, concerning signs or symptoms on history and physical, or recent changes in pulmonary status.

Cardiovascular

The most common serious perioperative complications stem from cardiovascular events. It has been noted in the literature that up to 5% of patients undergoing noncardiac surgery will develop a major cardiovascular complication perioperatively.[13] ECG should be obtained preoperatively on patients older than 50 years, particularly with a history of smoking, or any patients with symptoms or signs on history or physical examination of cardiac conditions. Further cardiac testing is typically not required preoperatively. The American Heart Association/American College of Cardiology (AHA/ACC) guidelines from Fleisher and colleagues[13] recommend further testing for intermediate-risk and high-risk elective surgeries only if the patient has an active cardiac condition, such as decompensated heart failure, symptomatic or severe valvular disease, and has a poor functional status.

Hypertension is exceedingly common, affecting approximately 25% of all adults, and up to 70% of adults 70 years or older. End-organ damage is a significant concern in patients with longstanding hypertension, particularly if poorly controlled. This most frequently presents as ischemic heart disease, renal insufficiency, or cerebrovascular disease.[14] Although primary or essential hypertension is most common, workup should be pursued particularly in young otherwise healthy patients to rule out conditions such as hyperthyroidism, coarctation, or endocrine disorders, such as pheochromocytoma. In addition, it is important to rule out the use of anabolic steroids or illicit drugs (typically amphetamines), as they can complicate perioperative care as well.

There are multiple opinions with regard to hypertension and operative timing. However, Howell and colleagues[14] suggest delaying elective operations in the case of severe hypertension, which can be defined as a diastolic blood pressure (BP) >115 mm Hg or systolic BP >200 mm Hg. Once BP is less than 180/110 mm Hg and there is no end-organ damage associated, it is considered relatively safe to move forward; there is minimal evidence to suggest there is an association between a preoperative BP reading of 180/110 mm Hg or lower and cardiac risk. For patients beginning antihypertensive medications preoperatively, it should take 6 to 8 weeks or more to "normalize" their BP and avoid the significant cardiac or cerebral damage that can occur with rapid correction of chronic hypertension. This is why it is important to maintain a patient's BP near the baseline perioperatively, even if that is somewhat hypertensive. Chronic hypertension is associated with shifts in autoregulatory curves, making critical organs like the brain dependent on higher pressures for adequate blood flow.

In addition to hypertension, there are a number of other risk factors for cardiac disease, and one of the primary goals of the preoperative evaluation is the identification of such risks.[15] Coronary artery disease (CAD) can be asymptomatic and is estimated to go undiagnosed in 40% of men and 65% of women. Thus, identifiable risk factors for CAD are just as important as specific symptoms of CAD when evaluating patients. Risk factors include smoking, hypertension, older age, male sex, diabetes, and dyslipidemia. Although these traditional risk factors are important, they alone are not necessarily associated with an increased incidence of perioperative cardiac events. Comorbidities such as history of ischemic cardiac disease, congestive heart failure, renal insufficiency, cerebrovascular disease, diabetes, advanced age, and high-risk surgery are associated with increased perioperative adverse cardiac events. The Revised Cardiac Risk Index has been validated as a useful tool to stratify patients and predict adverse cardiac events in the perioperative period (**Table 3**).[16]

Heart failure

Heart failure affects approximately 2% of the population within the United States and carries with it considerable risk for morbidity and mortality perioperatively.[17] To further illustrate this, there is approximately a 5% risk of perioperative cardiac complications in the 50-year-old to 59-year-old demographic. However, this risk is increased to 20% to 30% in the same cohort with heart failure. Symptoms such as recent weight gain, shortness of breath, fatigue, dyspnea, orthopnea, and peripheral edema can clue the provider into a diagnosis of decompensated heart failure. Signs in the physical examination could include peripheral edema, ascites, hepatomegaly, jugular venous distention, third or fourth heart sounds, tachycardia, or rales. The New York Heart Association classification can prove useful to describe the severity of symptoms and is displayed in **Table 4**.[16]

Table 3 Revised cardiac risk index	
1. History of ischemic heart disease	No = 0; Yes = +1
2. History of congestive heart failure	No = 0; Yes = +1
3. History of cerebrovascular disease	No = 0; Yes = +1
4. History of diabetes requiring preoperative insulin use	No = 0; Yes = +1
5. Chronic kidney disease (creatinine >2 mg/dL)	No = 0; Yes = +1
6. Undergoing suprainguinal vascular, intraperitoneal, or intrathoracic surgery	No = 0; Yes = +1

Risk for cardiac event: Score of 0 = 0.4%, 1 = 1.0%, 2 = 2.4%, 3 or greater = >5.4%.
From Wijeysundera DJ, Swietzer B. Preoperative evaluation [Chapter 38]. In: Miller RD, editor. Miller's anesthesia. 8th edition. Philadelphia: Saunders Elsevier; 2015. p.1094; with permission.

Table 4
New York Heart Association (NYHA) heart failure classification

NYHA Class	Symptoms
I	Known cardiac disease but is asymptomatic, no limitations in ordinary physical activity.
II	Mild symptoms (mild shortness of breath and/or angina). Mild limitation during ordinary levels of activity.
III	Moderate limitation in activity secondary to symptoms with only minimal activity (walking short distance), only relief comes at rest.
IV	Severe limitations, symptomatic at rest.

From Wijeysundera DJ, Swietzer B. Preoperative evaluation [Chapter 38]. In: Miller RD, editor. Miller's anesthesia. 8th edition. Philadelphia: Saunders Elsevier; 2015. p. 1099; with permission.

A patient who is suspected of or known to suffer from heart failure requires a preoperative ECG, evaluation of electrolytes, blood urea nitrogen, creatinine, and possibly a brain natriuretic peptide (BNP). BNP is useful for a multitude of reasons in heart failure, including diagnosis, as well as prediction of adverse events in noncardiac cases. In decompensated heart failure, patients require hospital admission, echocardiogram, and when stabilized, cardiac stress testing. Referral of patients with heart failure to Cardiology for preoperative optimization is appropriate. Volume status will dictate the patient's pharmacologic needs on the operative date. Medical therapy includes beta-blockers, hydralazine, nitrates, and digoxin. Perioperatively, there is evidence that patients on beta-blockers should have them continued to minimize cardiac adverse events. In addition, patients potentially benefit long-term from angiotensin receptor blockers, angiotensin-converting enzyme inhibitors, diuretics, and antiplatelet therapy; however, these classes of medications should generally be held preoperatively. For those individuals in decompensated heart failure, it is prudent to postpone surgery when possible, and pursue further workup and treatment as described previously.

Aortic stenosis
Aortic stenosis is the most common valvular abnormality in adults older than 65 and affects up to 4% of individuals. Symptoms associated with aortic stenosis include angina, heart failure, syncope and often dyspnea with exertion. A newfound systolic ejection murmur is suspicious of aortic stenosis and requires an ECG. Likely findings include left ventricular hypertrophy, ST-T wave changes, left axis deviation, or left bundle branch block.[18] If the ECG is abnormal or the patient demonstrates the symptoms described, an echocardiogram is recommended. An activated partial thromboplastin time (aPTT) should be evaluated with laboratory tests as well. Some patients with severe aortic stenosis develop acquired von Willebrand syndrome as a result of the turbulent blood flow, and may be prone to bleeding.

From an anesthesia standpoint, severe aortic stenosis poses a major risk for perioperative myocardial infarction and arrest. This makes induction of general anesthesia and emergence particularly high risk, and these patients require close hemodynamic monitoring, often with an arterial line before induction. Unfortunately, neuraxial anesthesia also poses a major risk in these patients due to the profound sympathectomy and reduction in preload and afterload. Postoperatively, these patients should be closely monitored, with careful attention to maintain euvolemia, normal sinus rhythm, and avoid hypotension. Atrial fibrillation or tachyarrhythmias are poorly tolerated with severe aortic stenosis. Given the risk associated and complexity of these patients, elective podiatric surgery may be postponed to pursue valvuloplasty or valve replacement to mitigate some of the cardiac risk if symptomatic, severe, or critical aortic stenosis is present. This highlights the importance of involving specialists before the operative day.

Antiplatelet and anticoagulant management

Perioperative management of antiplatelet and anticoagulant medications is an increasingly complex topic given the many newer classes of medications, lack of reliable reversal agents, and laboratory testing for many drugs, variable drug half-lives, and the wide range of indications for patients to be on these medications. For each procedure, it is necessary to weigh the risk of bleeding with the risk of discontinuing antiplatelet or anticoagulation therapy. If the risk of both is relatively high, a shorter-acting, reversible drug, such as heparin, can be used as a bridging agent.[19]

Those at highest risk for a thrombotic event include individuals with a history of a mechanical heart valve, transient ischemic attacks or stroke, venous thromboembolism (VTE) in the past 3 to 12 months, or an inherited thrombophilia, including protein C, S, or antithrombin deficiency, and antiphospholipid antibodies. Other major risk factors include atrial fibrillation, diabetes, congestive heart failure, age older than 75, active cancer, pregnancy, and hypertension. Atrial fibrillation alone is a moderate risk factor for perioperative thrombotic complications.[20]

Spyropoulos and Douketis[21] stratified surgical bleeding risk into 2 categories: high bleeding risk and low bleeding risk. These are defined by a 2-day risk of major bleed being between 2% to 4% or 0% to 2%, respectively. Many foot surgeries can be classified in a high bleeding risk category.[21] Omran and colleagues[22] developed a scoring system based on patient risk factors known as HAS-BLED. HAS-BLED stands for hypertension, abnormal renal or liver function, stroke, bleeding tendency, labile international normalized ratios, elderly age, and antiplatelet drugs or alcohol. All of these are associated with higher rates of perioperative bleeding.

There is no scoring scheme or classification system that can be used to determine with certainty whether or not to stop anticoagulation preoperatively. Generally, this decision should be made in conjunction with the other physicians caring for the patient and is based on clinical judgment. In those scheduled for elective surgery with high bleeding risk but also elevated risk of thromboembolic event (VTE), surgery should be postponed until their risk of VTE is minimized as much as possible. In all patients, aspirin should be continued perioperatively if possible, and home antiplatelet or anticoagulant medication regimens should be resumed as soon as reasonably safe postoperatively. When this time frame is unclear, involvement of consult services such as vascular medicine or cardiology can help to weigh the risks of holding versus restarting these medications. Sometimes, such as in patients with recent VTE, temporary vena cava filters are used while off anticoagulation.

One circumstance in which there is clear evidence regarding continuation of medications is related to coronary stents. Due to the high risk of in-stent thrombosis, which is associated with high mortality, dual antiplatelet therapy is recommended for a minimum of 2 weeks after angioplasty, 1 month after bare metal stents, and 1 year after drug-eluting stents. Elective surgery requiring stopping aspirin or other antiplatelet agents should be postponed until after this time frame and aspirin should always be continued if possible.

In patients at higher risk of VTE on chronic anticoagulation that must be stopped preoperatively, bridging with heparin can be used to minimize the time without anticoagulation. Heparin is short acting and reversible with protamine, making it a good choice.[23–25] Other anticoagulants have longer half-lives and more complex or no reversal agents. Coumadin typically must be held for 5 days preoperatively. For emergent surgery, effects of coumadin can be addressed with fresh frozen plasma, prothrombin complex concentrates, or vitamin K if time allows. Clopidogrel is a common antiplatelet drug that also is typically held for 5 days. There is no reliable reversal agent for this drug. Similarly, most of the other newer anticoagulants have no reversal agents; however, recently, the monoclonal antibody idarucizumab was approved by the Food and Drug Administration for reversal of dabigatran. Because many of the anticoagulants affect factor or platelet function rather than levels, laboratory studies of coagulation may be normal and not reflect their action. In emergent situations, specialized blood tests such as thromboelastography can be used to accurately evaluate a patient's coagulation status.

Diabetes

Diabetes has become a significant burden on the US medical system. The Centers for Disease Control and Prevention reports that more than 29 million people, or approximately 9.3% of the US population, suffer from the disease. Podiatry plays an important role in the management of these patients and diabetic individuals often make up most of a podiatrist's practice. It is important to understand the disease and the differences between type 1 and type 2 diabetes. In addition, there are significant comorbidities, both microvascular and macrovascular, that are a direct result of the disease process. Neuropathy, nephropathy, CAD, cerebrovascular disease, and large vessel disease are all common in diabetic individuals.

The effects of diabetes on the cardiovascular system cannot be understated. Diabetic patients should automatically be considered intermediate risk for major perioperative cardiac complications. For comparison, this would be at a level consistent with exertional angina or a history of myocardial infarction.[13,26] Additional risk factors that can clue a provider in on increased cardiac risk in the diabetic cohort are autonomic neuropathy, erectile dysfunction, uncontrolled hyperglycemia, and the duration of the disease. Myocardial infarction is often silent in diabetic individuals due to neuropathy.

Chronic kidney disease is discussed in more detail, but it is worth mentioning here as it is common among diabetic patients. Nearly half of the US population on dialysis is diabetic. When you add in hypertension and advanced age (>55 years old), that accounts for nearly 90% of patients suffering from renal insufficiency. Screening for renal insufficiency is an accepted practice in diabetic individuals, as patients often do not become symptomatic until the disease state is far progressed. Preoperative ECG is necessary given that diabetes is a CAD equivalent. In addition, it is important to evaluate the electrolyte profile preoperatively.

Preoperative workup should evaluate the adequacy of glycemic control, their current drug regimen, and whether neuropathy, nephropathy, CAD, or other comorbidities have developed as a result of their disease. Hemoglobin A1c (HgA1c) is the best measure of glycemic control, as this is independent of fasting state and reflects several months of glucose control. The American Diabetes Association recommends a HgA1c of less than 7% as an optimal target. Dronge and colleagues[27] reported a significant increase in rates of infection in diabetic individuals undergoing major noncardiac surgery when their HgA1c was greater than 7%.[28,29] A retrospective analysis by Abdelmalak and colleagues[30] showed a significant difference in 1-year mortality based on blood glucose; 3% to 5% incidence of mortality at 1 year in those with a preoperative blood glucose of 60 to 100 mg/dL compared with 12% with blood glucose greater than 216 mg/dL. Finally Han and Kang[31] noted that there is a significantly increased risk of wound development in individuals with a HgA1c >8%. It is obvious that optimizing blood glucose control preoperatively has profound effects on outcome and should be a priority, especially in elective surgery. Perioperative medication dosing for diabetic individuals per ASA guidelines includes discontinuing all fast-acting insulin on the day of surgery and administering only half of the basal insulin the night before surgery. Oral hypoglycemic medications, particularly metformin and sulfonylureas, should be held for surgery due to the risk of lactic acidosis and hypoglycemia, respectively.

Renal Disease

Chronic kidney disease (CKD) is defined as a decreased glomerular filtration rate (GFR), less than 60 mL/min for at least 3 months or significant proteinuria. Once a patient has a GFR that has declined to less than 15 mL/min it is classified as chronic renal failure. Acute renal failure can be defined by several criteria, including a decrease in urine output to less than 0.5 mL/kg per hour or an increase in creatinine by 0.3 or greater than 50% increase. Finally, end-stage renal disease (ESRD) is loss of renal function for 3 or more months.[16]

As mentioned in prior sections, CKD is closely associated with comorbidities such as hypertension and diabetes. It also represents a significant risk factor for CAD. Annually, approximately 8% of patients with ESRD die of cardiac events. Preoperative creatinine of 2.0 mg/dL or higher is a criterion to prompt cardiac workup, particularly for intermediate-risk and high-risk surgery, per AHA/ACC guidelines. Pericardial effusions, pericarditis, diastolic and systolic heart failure, as well as valvular heart disease secondary to calcification are common in dialysis patients.[32]

Anemia is also common in patients with renal disease due to erythropoietin deficiency. Aggressive therapy with exogenous erythropoietin is sometimes used preoperatively; however, this has led to complications with increased morbidity and vascular events and is not currently recommended.[33] Do not be fooled by a normal platelet count, platelet dysfunction is a well-known complication of CKD causing increased bleeding complications despite a normal platelet count, prothrombin time, and aPTT.[34,35] Desmopressin can sometimes be helpful if bleeding complications do occur.

Electrolyte and calcium abnormalities, hypoalbuminemia, and hypercholesterolemia are common in CKD as well. Preoperative testing should include an electrolyte panel, with potassium checked on the day of surgery, and an ECG. Common findings can include left ventricular hypertrophy, peaked t waves secondary to hyperkalemia, flattened t waves, and prolonged PR and QT intervals secondary to hypokalemia. Further testing with echocardiogram should be pursued if there are significant ECG abnormalities or concerning signs or symptoms on history or physical examination.[36,37] In patients on dialysis, it is essential to coordinate the timing of dialysis with the operative day. Ideally, patients should be dialyzed within 24 hours of surgery. However, careful monitoring and management of electrolytes and volume status is critical postoperatively.

PREOPERATIVE DIAGNOSTIC STUDIES

The recommendations for preoperative diagnostic testing are a topic of ongoing debate. Current expert opinion suggests there is no need for standardized preoperative testing regardless of age or medical comorbidities, as it is exceedingly expensive, upward of $4 billion a year in the United States. With the standard model of preoperative planning, there is significant inefficiency and potential for misdiagnosis secondary to false-positive or borderline test results requiring additional treatment and testing.[38] There are no concrete or steadfast guidelines with regard to preanesthesia diagnostic testing. However, in 2002 the ASA published recommendations that testing and consultation be done only on the basis of a reasonable expectation that the patient may have an abnormal value and that such a value will affect whether to proceed with surgery or how to provide perioperative care.[39] **Table 5** summarizes some recommendations for preoperative testing depending on comorbidities. Communication between the anesthesia and surgical teams is the best approach to preoperative testing, as no accepted standard exists after an exhaustive literature review.

It is important to note that **Table 5** is simply recommendations or guidelines as to a starting point with respect to a preoperative diagnostic evaluation. As an example, a relationship between renal disease and cardiac disease is discussed. In **Table 5**, which comes from a prominent anesthesiology textbook, there is no recommendation for a preoperative ECG in patients with renal disease. It is more than reasonable to order an ECG in the face of potential surgery and a patient with renal disease. Every preoperative evaluation should be individualized and not just indiscriminately ordered based solely on any set of guidelines.

CONSIDERATIONS IN LOWER EXTREMITY ANESTHESIA

Although the final decision regarding choice of anesthesia falls on the anesthesiologist, it is necessary for podiatric surgeons to have a basic understanding of anesthetic options and their distinct advantages and disadvantages. There are 4 basic types of anesthesia: general, MAC, neuraxial, and regional anesthesia. Operative needs and patient factors determine which of these options is reasonable and safe to consider.

General anesthesia consists of a hypnosis, unconsciousness, amnesia, analgesia, and immobility or muscle relaxation, providing the most predictable and stable surgical field. This is generally achieved with a combination of medications given intravenously and inhaled. The tradeoff is that general anesthesia is usually accompanied by significant hemodynamic and respiratory changes, especially during induction and emergence periods, requiring constant monitoring and frequent intervention by anesthesia providers. These changes can be particularly profound in patients with significant underlying cardiopulmonary disease, who have an increased risk of requiring prolonged postoperative mechanical ventilation or perioperative vasopressor use. Also, most of the anesthetic drugs depend on renal and/or hepatic clearance, which is of importance in patients with impaired liver or kidney function at baseline who can have prolonged drug effects.

MAC involves the administration of a sedative, anxiolytic, and/or analgesic medication while under the direct, constant care of an anesthesia provider. Generally, it consists of a deep level of sedation; however, preparation is always made for general anesthesia should it be required. MAC is typically accompanied by regional or local anesthesia to provide surgical-level analgesia. The benefit of MAC compared with general anesthesia is that it less frequently requires endotracheal intubation or airway manipulation, and postoperative recovery from anesthesia is faster. However, because there is no muscle relaxation and the patient is not deeply anesthetized, the surgical field is less predictable and there can be movement and patient interaction during the procedure. In addition, patients who have difficulty lying flat or positioning for surgery, may not tolerate MAC even if the procedure otherwise lends itself to that anesthetic technique. The same can be said for those with significant respiratory disease or a difficult airway; administration of sedative drugs with respiratory depression may make general anesthesia with a definitive airway a safer option in these patients.

Neuraxial anesthesia consists of spinal or epidural anesthesia and is provided by a single injection or continuous infusion of local anesthetic. These techniques can

Table 5
Recommendations for preoperative testing depending on comorbidities

Preoperative Diagnosis	ECG	Chest Radiograph	Hct/Hb	CBC	Electrolytes	Creatinine	Glucose	Coagulation	LFTs	Drug Levels	Ca
Cardiac disease	—	—	—	—	—	—	—	—	—	—	—
History of MI	X	—	—	X	±	—	—	—	—	—	—
Chronic stable angina	X	±	—	X	±	—	—	—	—	—	—
CHF	X	±	—	—	—	—	—	—	—	—	—
HTN	X	±	—	—	X[a]	X	—	—	—	—	—
Chronic atrial fibrillation	X	—	—	—	—	—	—	—	—	X[b]	—
PAD	X	—	—	—	—	—	—	—	—	—	—
Valvular heart disease	X	±	—	—	—	—	—	—	—	—	—
Pulmonary disease	—	—	—	—	—	—	—	—	—	—	—
COPD	X	±	—	X	—	—	—	—	—	X[c]	—
Asthma	(PFTs only if symptomatic; otherwise no tests required)										
Diabetes	X	—	—	—	±	X	X	—	—	—	—
Liver disease	—	—	—	—	—	—	—	—	—	—	—
Infectious hepatitis	—	—	—	—	—	—	—	X	X	—	—
Alcohol or drug-induced hepatitis	—	—	—	—	—	—	—	X	X	—	—
Tumor infiltration	—	—	—	—	—	—	—	X	X	—	—
Renal disease	—	—	X	—	X	X	—	—	—	—	—
Hematologic disorders	—	—	—	X	—	—	—	—	—	—	—
Coagulopathies	—	—	—	X	—	—	—	X	—	—	—
CNS disorders	—	—	—	—	—	—	—	—	—	—	—
Stroke	X	—	—	X	X	—	X	—	—	X	—
Seizures	X	—	—	X	X	—	X	—	—	X	—

Condition / Drug therapy													
Tumor	X	—	—	—	—	—	—	—	—	—	—	—	X
Vascular disorders or aneurysms	X	—	—	—	—	—	—	—	—	—	—	X	—
Malignant disease	—	—	—	—	—	—	—	—	—	—	—	—	—
Hyperthyroidism	X	—	X	X	X	—	—	—	—	—	—	—	X
Hypothyroidism	X	—	X	X	X	X	X	—	—	—	—	—	—
Cushing disease	—	—	X	X	X	X	—	X	—	—	—	—	—
Addison disease	—	—	X	X	X	X	—	X	—	—	—	—	—
Hyperparathyroidism	X	—	X	X	X	—	—	—	X	—	—	—	X
Hypoparathyroidism	X	—	X	X	X	—	—	—	—	—	—	—	X
Morbid obesity	X	±	—	—	X	X	—	—	X	—	—	—	—
Malabsorption or poor nutrition	X	X	X	X	X	X	X	—	—	—	—	—	—
Select drug therapies	—	—	—	—	—	—	—	—	—	—	—	—	—
Digoxin (digitalis)[b]	X	—	—	—	X	—	—	—	—	—	—	±	X
Anticoagulants	—	X	—	X	—	—	X	—	—	—	—	—	—
Phenytoin (Dilantin)	—	—	—	—	—	—	—	—	—	—	—	—	X
Phenobarbital	—	—	—	—	—	—	—	—	—	—	—	X	X
Diuretics[a]	—	—	X	X	X	—	—	—	—	—	—	—	—
Corticosteroids	—	—	X	—	X	—	—	X	—	—	—	—	—
Chemotherapy	—	±	X	—	X	—	—	X	—	X	—	—	—
Aspirin or NSAIDs	—	—	—	—	—	—	—	—	—	—	—	—	—
Theophylline[c]	—	—	—	—	—	—	—	—	—	—	X	—	X

^a If the patient is taking diuretics.
^b If the patient is taking digoxin.
^c If the patient is taking theophylline.

Abbreviations: ±, consider this test, but not firmly recommended; Ca, calcium; CBC, complete blood count; CHF, congestive heart failure; CNS, central nervous system; COPD, chronic obstructive pulmonary disease; ECG, electrocardiogram; Hb, hemoglobin; Hct, hematocrit; HTN, hypertension; LFTs, liver function tests; MI, myocardial infarction; NSAID, nonsteroidal antiinflammatory drug; PAD, peripheral arterial disease; PFT, pulmonary function test; X, obtain.

From Wijeysundera DJ, Sweitzer B. Preoperative evaluation [Chapter 38]. In: Miller RD, editor. Miller's anesthesia. 8th edition. Philadelphia: Saunders Elsevier; 2015. p. 1142; with permission.

provide good anesthesia and analgesia for lower extremity procedures. As cervical and thoracic coverage is not required, there is minimal respiratory effect, making it a good choice in patients with significant respiratory disease. Due to the risk of hematoma and neurologic damage, this technique is not an option in those with coagulopathy or on antiplatelet or anticoagulant medication that has not been held appropriately preoperatively.[40] Additionally, those with significant cardiac disease, aortic stenosis, or hypertrophic cardiomyopathy are at risk for complications secondary to the profound sympathectomy and decrease in preload that occurs with neuraxial anesthesia. Other rare but potentially serious complications of this technique include spinal cord injury, infection, or local anesthetic toxicity.

Which is best for your patients, general or neuraxial anesthesia? According to Basques and colleagues,[41] there is no significant benefit or risk of one over the other when either would be appropriate. Potential benefits of neuraxial anesthesia include apparent decreased rates of deep vein thrombosis, pulmonary embolism, postoperative ileus, and lower amounts of postoperative narcotic use.[42] There is also some evidence that neuraxial anesthesia may decrease rates of cancer recurrence compared with general anesthesia.[43–48] A potential drawback of neuraxial anesthesia compared with general is that it may slightly prolong total operating room time, depending on the anesthetic provider.

Regional anesthesia or peripheral nerve blocks are of exceptional benefit in podiatric surgery, either as a stand-alone surgical anesthetic or in conjunction with another technique for intraoperative and postoperative pain control. The use of regional blocks can significantly reduce opioid requirements. Most commonly, the popliteal block is used, along with a saphenous nerve block to provide complete analgesia for the lower leg and foot. As with neuraxial techniques, some caution must be used with patients on blood thinning medications or coagulopathy. Other potential risks include infection and local anesthetic toxicity. When used for surgical anesthesia, most patients will require MAC in conjunction with regional anesthesia or peripheral nerve blocks.

SUMMARY

Preoperative assessment and perioperative care of podiatric patients is exceedingly complex. In today's health climate, an impetus has been placed on the need for cost-effective care. A standard preoperative protocol should be avoided and individualized care used to decrease financial strain on the medical system and unnecessary testing. A team approach involving communication with the patient, surgeon, anesthesia team, primary care physician, and appropriate specialists is necessary to provide optimal care and achieve the best possible surgical outcomes. All patients should undergo a detailed preoperative history and physical examination, after which it can be determined whether additional diagnostic tests and consults are needed. This review is by no means comprehensive, but provides a foundation for some important considerations in the podiatric surgical candidate.

REFERENCES

1. Hurwitz E, Simon M, Vinta SR, et al. Adding examples to the ASA-physical status classification improves correct assignment to patients. Anesthesiology 2017; 126(4):614–22.
2. Owens WD, Felts JA, Spitznagel EL Jr. ASA physical status classifications: a study of consistency of ratings. Anesthesiology 1978;49:239–43.
3. Fleisher LA, Pasternak LR, Herbert R, et al. Inpatient hospital admission and death after outpatient surgery in elderly patients. Arch Surg 2004;139:67–72.

4. Girish M, Trayner E, Dammann O, et al. Symptom-limited stair climbing as a predictor of postoperative complications after high-risk surgery. Chest 2001;120: 1147–51.

5. Chung F, Yegneswaran B, Liao P. STOP questionnaire: a tool to screen patients for obstructive sleep apnea. Anesthesiology 2008;108:812–21.

6. Katz I, Stradling J, Slutsjy AS, et al. Do patients with obstructive sleep apnea have thick necks? Am Rev Respir Dis 1990;141:1228–31.

7. Brooks-Brunn JA. Predictors of postoperative pulmonary complications following abdominal surgery. Chest 1997;111:564.

8. British Thoracic Society; Society of Cardiothoracic Surgeons of Great Britain and Ireland Working Party. BTS guidelines: guidelines on the selection of patients with lung cancer for surgery. Thorax 2001;56:89.

9. Brunelli A, Kim AW, Berger KI, et al. Physiologic evaluation of the patient with lung cancer being considered for resectional surgery: diagnosis and management of lung cancer, 3rd ed: American College of Chest Physicians evidence-based clinical practice guidelines. Chest 2013;143:e166s.

10. Qaseem A, Snow V, Fitterman N, et al. Risk assessment for and strategies to reduce perioperative pulmonary complications for patients undergoing noncardiothoracic surgery: a guideline from the American College of Physicians. Ann Intern Med 2006;144:575.

11. Archer C, Levy AR, McGregor M. Value of routine preoperative chest x-rays: a meta-analysis. Can J Anaesth 1993;40:1022.

12. Rucker L, Frye EB, Staten MA. Usefulness of screening chest roentgenograms in preoperative patients. JAMA 1983;250:3209.

13. Fleisher LA, Beckman JA, Brown KA, et al. ACC/AHA 2006 guideline update on perioperative cardiovascular evaluation for noncardiac surgery: Focused update on perioperative beta-blocker therapy: a report of the American College of Cardiology/American Heart Association Task Force on Practice Guidelines. Circulation 2006;113:2662–74.

14. Howell SJ, Sear JW, Foex P. Hypertension, hypertensive heart disease and perioperative cardiac risk. Br J Anaesth 2004;92:570–83.

15. Van Klei WA, Bryson GL, Yang H, et al. The value of routine preoperative electrocardiography in predicting myocardial infarction after noncardiac surgery. Ann Surg 2007;246:165.

16. Wijeysundera DJ, Swietzer B. Chapter 38: preoperative evaluation. In: Miller RD, editor. Miller's anesthesia. 8th edition. Philadelphia: Saunders Elsevier; 2015. p. 1085–155.

17. Thom T, Haase N, Rosamond W, et al. Heart disease and stroke statistics subcommittee. Circulation 2006;113:e85–151.

18. Tashiro T, Pislaru SV, Blustin JM, et al. Perioperative risk of major non-cardiac surgery in patients with severe aortic stenosis: a reappraisal in contemporary practice. Eur Heart J 2014;35:2372.

19. Bell BR, Spyropoulos AC, Douketis JD. Perioperative management of the direct oral anticoagulants: a case-based review. Hematol Oncol Clin North Am 2016; 30:1073.

20. Douketis JD, Spyropoulos AC, Spencer FA, et al. Perioperative management of antithrombotic therapy: antithrombotic therapy and prevention of thrombosis, 9th ed: American College of Chest Physicians evidence-based clinical practice guidelines. Chest 2012;141:2012.

21. Spyropoulos AC, Douketis JD. How I treat anticoagulated patients undergoing an elective procedure or surgery. Blood 2012;120:2954.

22. Omran H, Bauersachs R, Rübenacker S, et al. The HAS-BLED score predicts bleedings during bridging of chronic oral anticoagulation. Results from the national multicentre BNK Online bRiDging REgistRy (BORDER). Thromb Haemost 2012;108:65.

23. Strebel N, Prins M, Agnelli G, et al. Preoperative or postoperative start of prophylaxis for venous thromboembolism with low-molecular-weight heparin in elective hip surgery? Arch Intern Med 2002;162:1451.

24. Levy JH, Tanaka KA, Dietrich W. Perioperative hemostatic management of patients treated with vitamin K antagonists. Anesthesiology 2008;109:918.

25. Douketis JD, Woods K, Foster GA, et al. Bridging anticoagulation with low-molecular-weight heparin after interruption of warfarin therapy is associated with a residual anticoagulant effect prior to surgery. Thromb Haemost 2005; 94:528.

26. Haffner SM, Lehto S, Ronnemaa T, et al. Mortality from coronary heart disease in subjects with type 2 diabetes and in nondiabetic subjects with and without prior myocardial infarction. N Engl J Med 1998;339:229–34.

27. Dronge AS, Perkal MF, Kancir S, et al. Long-term glycemic control and postoperative infectious complications. Arch Surg 2006;141:375–80 [discussion: 380].

28. Sato H, Carvalho G, Sato T, et al. The association of preoperative glycemic control, intraoperative insulin sensitivity, and outcomes after cardiac surgery. J Clin Endocrinol Metab 2010;95:4338.

29. Stryker LS, Abdel MP, Morrey ME, et al. Elevated postoperative blood glucose and preoperative hemoglobin A1C are associated with increased wound complications following total joint arthroplasty. J Bone Joint Surg Am 2013;95:808.

30. Abdelmalak BB, Knittel J, Abdelmalak JB, et al. Preoperative blood glucose concentrations and postoperative outcomes after elective non-cardiac surgery: an observational study. Br J Anaesth 2014;112:79–88.

31. Han HS, Kang SB. Relations between long-term glycemic control and postoperative wound and infectious complications after total knee arthroplasty in type 2 diabetics. Clin Orthop Surg 2013;5:118–23.

32. Straumann E, Meyer B, Misteli M, et al. Aortic and mitral valve disease in patients with end stage renal failure on long-term haemodialysis. Br Heart J 1992;67: 236–9.

33. Singh AK, Szczech L, Tang KL, et al. Correction of anemia with epoetin alfa in chronic kidney disease. N Engl J Med 2006;355:2085–98.

34. Boccardo P, Remuzzi G, Galbusera M. Platelet dysfunction in renal failure. Semin Thromb Hemost 2004;30:579–89.

35. Lindsay RM, Friesen M, Aronstam A, et al. Improvement of platelet function by increased frequency of hemodialysis. Clin Nephrol 1978;10:67.

36. Ahmed J, Weisberg LS. Hyperkalemia in dialysis patients. Semin Dial 2001; 14:348.

37. Esposito C, Bellotti N, Fasoli G, et al. Hyperkalemia-induced ECG abnormalities in patients with reduced renal function. Clin Nephrol 2004;62:465.

38. Johnson RK, Mortimer AJ. Routine pre-operative blood testing: is it necessary? Anaesthesia 2002;57:914–7.

39. American Society of Anesthesiologists Task Force on Preanesthesia Evaluation. Practice advisory for preoperative evaluation: a report by the American Society of Anesthesiologists task force on preanesthetic evaluation. Anesthesiology 2002;96:485–96.

40. Horlocker TT, Wedel DJ, Rowlingson JC, et al. Regional anesthesia in the patient receiving antithrombotic or thrombolytic therapy; American Society of Regional

Anesthesia and Pain Medicine evidence-based guidelines (third edition). Reg Anesth Pain Med 2010;35(1):64–101.

41. Basques BA, Bohl DD, Golinvaux NS, et al. General versus spinal anaesthesia for patients aged 70 years and older with a fracture of the hip. Bone Joint J 2015; 97-B:689.

42. Rodgers A, Walker N, Schug S, et al. Reduction of postoperative mortality and morbidity with epidural or spinal anaesthesia: results from overview of randomized trials. BMJ 2000;321:1493.

43. Sekandarzad MW, Van Zundert AAJ, Lirk PB, et al. Perioperative anesthesia care and tumor progression. Anesth Analg 2017;124:1697.

44. Aronson WL, McAuliffe MS, Miller K. Variability in the American Society of Anesthesiologists physical status scale. AANA J 2003;71:265–73.

45. Johnson RL, Kopp SL, Burkle CM, et al. Neuraxial vs general anaesthesia for total hip and total knee arthroplasty: a systematic review of comparative-effectiveness research. Br J Anaesth 2016;116:163.

46. Liu SS, Strodtbeck WM, Richman JM, et al. A comparison of regional versus general anesthesia for ambulatory anesthesia: a meta-analysis of randomized controlled trials. Anesth Analg 2005;101:1634.

47. Practice advisory for the prevention, diagnosis, and management of infectious complications associated with neuraxial techniques: an updated report by the American Society of Anesthesiologists task force on infectious complications associated with neuraxial techniques and the American Society of Regional Anesthesia and Pain Medicine. Anesthesiology 2017;126:585.

48. Lee KT, Park YU, Jegal H, et al. Femoral and sciatic nerve block for hindfoot and ankle surgery. J Orthop Sci 2014;19:546.

Prevention of Deep Venous Thromboembolism in Foot and Ankle Surgery

Preston Carr, MS[a], Duane J. Ehredt Jr, DPM[b,c,*], Alex Dawoodian, DPM[c]

KEYWORDS

- Thromboembolism • Chemoprophylaxis • Prophylaxis • Clot • Venous

KEY POINTS

- Despite low reported incidence rates, deep vein thrombosis (DVT) and pulmonary embolism (PE) remain a concern for foot and ankle surgeons.
- To date, there are no validated screening tools for venous thromboembolism (VTE) prophylaxis specifically following foot and ankle surgery.
- The consensus among most foot and ankle surgeons is that prophylaxis measures should be handled on a case-by-case basis.
- It is generally accepted that all nonpharmacologic prophylactic measures are used routinely, examples being reduction of modifiable risk factors or mechanoprophylaxis.
- When patients present with known risk factors (eg, previous VTE, oral contraceptive use, malignancy, Achilles surgery) most foot and ankle surgeons use pharmacologic prophylaxis measures.

INTRODUCTION

Throughout the medical community, the issue of discerning between prevention and treatment methods for deep vein thrombosis (DVT) can be daunting, considering the volume of information available in the literature. DVT is often accompanied mechanistically by pulmonary embolism (PE), and therefore when merged is referred to as venous thromboembolism (VTE). Lower extremity surgeons should have a working

Disclosure Statement: None.
[a] Kent State University College of Podiatric Medicine, 6000 Rockside Woods Boulevard, Independence, OH 44131, USA; [b] Division of Foot and Ankle Surgery, Kent State University College of Podiatric Medicine, 6000 Rockside Woods Boulevard, Independence, OH 44131, USA; [c] Podiatric Medicine and Surgery Residency Program, Saint Vincent Charity Medical Center, 2351 East 22nd Street, Cleveland, OH 44115, USA
* Corresponding author. Division of Foot and Ankle Surgery, Kent State University College of Podiatric Medicine, 6000 Rockside Woods Boulevard, Independence, OH 44131.
E-mail address: dehredt@kent.edu

knowledge regarding the clotting cascade (**Fig. 1**), as this will serve as the groundwork for understanding DVT formation, prophylaxis, and treatment. The danger of undiagnosed and untreated VTE can be a significant driving factor for long-term complications and morbidity, with the potential for mortality. Due to the possible chance of death, lower extremity surgeons must maintain a high index of suspicion for VTE.

DVT in foot and ankle surgery is often seen limited to the calf region and commonly associated with post-thrombotic syndrome (PTS) (**Fig. 2**), with occurrence rates of approximately 30% of total DVTs.[1,2] PTS is hallmarked by venous hypertension, which may cause pain, edema, hyperpigmentation, lipodermatosclerosis, dermatitis, and even frank ulceration. The routine use of prophylactic measures in foot and ankle surgery is not well understood. Various studies draw conclusions from differing populations and therefore recommendations for and against prophylaxis are often inconsistent. Recommendations range from injectable antithrombotic chemical prophylaxis to providing absolutely nothing but early range of motion.[3] Especially in the lower extremity, stratification of the risk factors involved in preoperative foot and ankle prophylaxis often involves extrapolation from similar validated methods found in the hip and knee literature. A variety of risk factors have been identified for VTE and include comorbidities such as diabetes mellitus, hypercholesterolemia, hypertension, tobacco use, active infection, cancer, increased age, obesity, previous history of VTE, oral contraception use, recent surgery, immobilization, and trauma (**Table 1**). Other hereditary conditions, such as factor V Leiden mutation, protein C and S, and antithrombin deficiencies also raise the probability of a VTE event. Appropriate identification of aforementioned acquired and inherited risks factors is mandated to limit patient exposure to VTE through appropriate risk factor–driven prophylactic measures. Outside consultation is warranted in the setting of hereditary risk factors and the

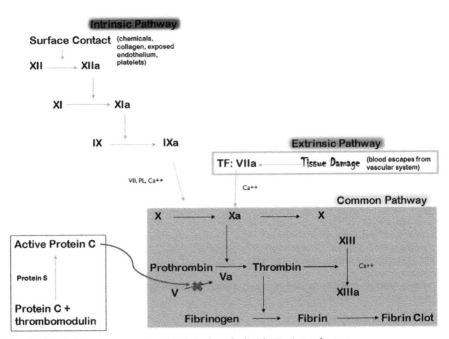

Fig. 1. The clotting cascade. PL, platelet phospholipid; TF, tissue factor.

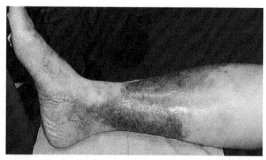

Fig. 2. PTS of the right lower extremity. Note in this case the post-phlebitic hyperpigmentation, edema, and lipodermatosclerosis changes consistent with PTS.

need to treat foot and ankle pathology via nonoperative immobilization or surgery with or without postoperative immobilization.

The exact incidence rate of DVT formation following foot and ankle surgery is also unknown. Published rates have been as low as 0.22% and as high as 38.5% following Achilles surgery.[3,4] Due to the infinite combinations of potential absolute and modifiable risk factors, validated DVT prophylaxis guidelines following foot and ankle surgery have yet to materialize. We believe that a more uniform approach needs to be followed to minimize the risk of VTE formation and its sequelae, while also mitigating the unnecessary use of chemoprophylactic agents. To achieve this, clinicians must be well versed in identifying patients at risk for DVT formation, and the appropriate interventions necessary to prevent this potentially disastrous complication. This article summarizes pathophysiological forces that drive VTE development, lists the absolute and modifiable risk factors, and reviews the currently available prophylactic strategies available to the foot and ankle surgeon.

HEMODYNAMICS AND PATHOLOGY

Lower extremity DVT often results from an impaired venous return, endothelial injury, or dysfunction and hypercoagulability. Specifically, Virchow postulated a triad of

Table 1	
Known risk factors for deep venous thrombosis formation	
Acquired Risk Factors	**Inherited Risk Factors**
Elevated body mass index	Antiphospholipid antibody syndrome
Cancer and treatments (within 6 mo)	
Tobacco use	Factor V Leiden mutation
Hypertension	Protein C or S deficiency
Hyperlipidemia	Prothrombin gene mutation
Diabetes mellitus	
Limb immobilization	Elevated Factor VIII
Pregnancy or oral contraceptive/hormone replacement therapy	Antithrombin deficiency
Previous venous thromboembolism	
Recent surgery	
Recent trauma	
Prolonged air travel	
Use of general anesthesia	
Tourniquet use	

hemodynamic causes for DVT; the issue of stasis, which obstructs antegrade and retrograde velocity through certain valves, changes in venous wall composition (possibly due to primary disease), and changes in blood composition and coaguability.[5] It is important to note that the idea of thrombosis and hemostasis is based on the concept that the processes are localized (specifically in the calf region for this article). Simply altering the postulations without specification (ie, popliteal vein) will only lead to widespread thrombin generation and immediate intravascular dissemination.

Postsurgical trauma and stasis are initiating factors that contribute to the activation of the innate clotting cascade of the lower extremity. Hemostasis is a normal and necessary introduction into the healing of bodily tissues following surgical introduction. This system is kept in check by several antithrombotic mechanisms. There are 3 major natural anticoagulant pathways: the heparin-antithrombin pathway, the protein C anticoagulant pathway, and the tissue factor inhibitor pathway. Of these, defects in antithrombin, and each of the components of the protein C anticoagulant pathway, are associated with increased risks of thrombotic disease in humans (protein S, thrombomodulin, and possibly Endothelial Protein C Receptor [EPCR]).[5–10] In the lower extremity, this is usually localized in the venous soleus sinusoids and cusps of the valves, typically confirmed through direct autopsy and phlebography.[1,5,11–13] The patient may present with a positive Homan sign, which is pain in the calf on dorsiflexion of the ankle, and/or swelling of the affected limb, and is commonly thought to be clinical evidence of a calf DVT.[1] The valves are avascular, which, in combination with lack of oxygenated blood in veins, stresses the surrounding endothelium into a hypoxemic state. This hypoxemia induces Hypoxia-Inducible Factor 1 (HIF1) and Early-Growth-Response Protein 1 (EGRP1), in conjunction with the production of a reactive oxygen species, inducing upregulation of endothelial proteins.[14] This state causes an increase in hematocrit leading to a hypercoagulable environment.[5] In addition, the activated surrounding endothelium increases expression of procoagulation proteins, such as Tissue Factor 21, cytokines, and specific surface adhesion molecules that promote recruitment and leukocyte adhesion, in essence initiating a thrombus.[15] The pathology of the clot works through Tissue Factor, which leads to initiation and amplification phases and the proliferation of the cascade.

Many of the anticoagulant pathways are triggered by endothelial cell surface components, including thrombomodulin, EPCR, tissue factor pathway inhibitor, and heparinlike proteoglycans. EPCR and thrombin bound to thrombomodulin initiate the protein C pathway responsible for the inactivation of critical cofactors Va and VIIIa, tissue factor pathway inhibitor blocks tissue factor–initiated coagulation and heparinlike proteoglycans stimulate antithrombin's inhibitor activity toward coagulation enzymes like thrombin. Therefore, as the blood moves from the larger vessels into the microcirculation, the efficacy of the natural anticoagulants increases dramatically, in large part because of the vastly greater endothelial cell area exposed to blood in the capillaries compared with the major arteries or veins.[5,16,17] This may, in part, explain the relatively low VTE rate in foot and ankle surgery.

If a clot forms and does not resolve, the venous thrombi will remain static in the popliteal or femoral system of the calf and thigh, respectively. The clot will eventually undergo thrombolysis and recanalization. Those that break free, and embolize, will follow antegrade flow back to the heart, eventually lodging into the pulmonary vascular tree. Furthermore, the platelets produced in the cascade secrete potent mediators for pulmonary vasoconstriction (ie, histamine and serotonin), which result in bronchoconstriction. Bronchoconstriction leads to immediate alveolar hypoxemia, causing decreased perfusion of the distal alveoli, increased minute ventilation/respiratory alkalosis, hypocapnia and ultimately increased pulmonary vascular resistance.[18,19] Hemodynamic effects are multifold. The hematocrit occlusion's effect on pulmonary vascular resistance increases right ventricular afterload, dilation, and hypertrophy, which clinically correlates to a "parasternal heave" and a loud P2 (pulmonic valve closure) sound on cardiac auscultation. If the occlusion continues to render significant blockage, the forward flow of the heart to the left side is reduced (decreased ventricular filling), eventually the patient will experience heart failure, shock, and death.[18,19]

MECHANICAL VERSUS CHEMICAL PROPHYLAXIS OF DEEP VEIN THROMBOSIS SPECIFIC TO FOOT AND ANKLE SURGERY

The attempt to standardize treatment and prophylaxis in VTE following foot and ankle surgery has been difficult. The current literature on prevention sheds some insight into the efficacy of each method. Almost all investigators recommend initiating this process with patient education and comprehension. Every foot and ankle surgeon should incorporate VTE statistics, physiology, and early warning signs as part of the surgical consultation and routine. It is believed that patient education drives compliance, and may possibly aid in early diagnosis should DVT occur. Nonetheless, the controversy as to when formal prophylaxis should be administered, and what that method consists of, remains an issue for preoperative foot and ankle protocols. Established in 2010, the National Institute for Health and Care Excellence (NICE) guidelines called for VTE prophylaxis to consist of pharmacologic thromboprophylaxis in all patients with lower limb trauma and/or surgery who are immobilized in a plaster cast along with other indications.[20] Likewise, the American College of Chest Physicians (ACCP) recommends the use of chemical prophylaxis or an intermittent pneumatic compression device (**Fig. 3**) for patients undergoing major orthopedic surgery in their latest 2012 guidelines.[21] However, surveys of the current practice of foot and ankle surgeons present inconsistencies and lack of firm recommendations for a mechanical or chemical intervention.

Mechanical prophylaxis is simply external, physical devices that can be categorized as elastic compression stockings (**Fig. 4**) and successive compression calf pumps or foot pumps on the contralateral extremity. These devices can be used both intraoperatively and postoperatively.[22,23] Elasticated compression devices help to prevent DVT by applying a varying amount of pressure to different parts of the lower limb. This

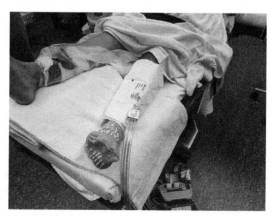

Fig. 3. Sequential compression device on the nonoperative limb. This form of prophylaxis is almost always used by foot and ankle surgeons.

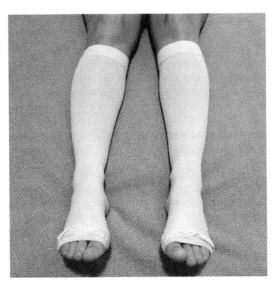

Fig. 4. Thromboembolic deterrent (TED) hose on a female patient. TED hose provides gradual compression from distal to proximal, and is an excellent modality for both the surgical and nonsurgical limb. In this case, TED hose is applied to the surgical limb at the first dressing change (approximately 10 days postoperative).

allows for a "milking" effect of the limb and thereby reduces venous stasis. A Cochrane review from 2014 demonstrated that mechanical prophylaxis devices reduced the incidence of DVT from 26% to 13%, as compared with control groups.[24] The utility and efficacy of these methods have not been related, or extrapolated as statistically similar to chemoprophylaxis, but the complications are negligible, which is appealing to surgeons and patients alike. On the other hand, the more commonly used method of chemical or pharmacologic prophylaxis includes the use of anticoagulants, such as warfarin, antiplatelets such as aspirin, unfractionated heparin, and low molecular weight heparin (LMWH). Chemical prophylaxis does have risks, ranging from bruising and minor surgical wound complications to possible major bleeding leading to significant morbidity and even mortality. Unique to the delicate soft tissue envelope of the foot and ankle, anticoagulation may substantially increase local complications associated with wound drainage and hematoma. Additionally, heparin carries the risk of heparin-induced thrombocytopenia, which is a complication that can lead to PE, ischemia, stroke, and myocardial infarction.[22,23]

Hemodynamics tells us that veins are thinner-walled distensible vessels, and due to the nature of gravity, blood tends to pool in the feet and legs. This vessel distension can cause varicose veins, leading to slower velocity and increased risk of thrombus formation. General anesthesia blocks voluntary skeletal muscle contraction, resulting in mechanical loss of the pressure volume relationship of venous return to the heart. The idea of mechanical prophylaxis is based on the principle of contraction mimicry to compress the venous system and assist venous return. Considering the low cost, commendable efficacy, and minimal to no adverse effects, the authors recommend using mechanical prophylactic measures for all lower extremity surgical patients. The senior author (DJE) of this article routinely uses sequential compression devices immediately on the contralateral limb before, during, and after the surgical procedure. Postoperatively, the surgical limb is always addressed with a multilayer Jones compression dressing and TED (thromboembolic disease) hose routinely used on the contralateral limb until ambulation is initiated.

The use of chemical prophylaxis is seemingly a common standard of practice for foot and ankle surgeons, despite a controversial risk-benefit scenario of consequential bleeding in the patients ultimately leading to VTE. The most common anticoagulant pharmacologic agents available to combat VTE are warfarin, LMWH, aspirin, low-dose unfractionated heparin (LDUH), rivaroxaban, and dabigatran. These drugs and prophylactic dosages are listed in **Table 2**. Warfarin is a vitamin K antagonist that is cheap and readily available. Although easily obtained, warfarin does require active monitoring by the prescriber. Surgeons must monitor prothrombin time (international normalized ratio [INR] goal of 2–3) and any warfarin regimen should be stopped in patients at least 3 days before surgery or an unnecessary hypercoagulable state can result from the inhibition of protein C, a critical clotting cascade intermediate.[25,26] Aspirin (acetylsalicylic acid) is also a cheap, readily available agent, but its irreversible cyclooxygenase inhibitor activity is associated with high risk of gastrointestinal bleeding and relative drug-drug interactions. When either agent is used in combination therapy, the relative risks of gastrointestinal bleeding are exacerbated.[25] The LDUH and LMWH agents target the initiation stage of the clotting factor cascade and are classified as an antithrombin III activator and Factor Xa inhibitor, respectively. In a warfarin regimen that ceases 2 to 3 days before surgery, LDUH can bridge the presurgery gap and provide a cheap, parenterally administered, low bleeding risk, method of antithrombosis. LMWH provides an efficacious antifibrin clot inhibition that involves subcutaneous administration with minimal potential for heparin-induced thrombocytopenia. Enoxaparin does, however, carry the potential injection site hematoma complication.[25,26]

Table 2
Commonly prescribed chemoprophylactic agents with recommended prophylactic dosages

Drug	Mechanism of Action	Prophylactic Dosage
Warfarin	Inhibits the vitamin K–dependent synthesis of biologically active forms of the calcium-dependent clotting factors II, VII, IX, and X, as well as the regulatory factors protein C, protein S, and protein Z.	2–5 mg PO daily. Target INR 2–3. Consider 4 wk of therapy if immobilized.
Aspirin (acetylsalicylic acid)	Cyclooxygenase inhibitor. Decreases prostaglandin and thromboxane synthesis, thereby inhibiting platelet aggregation.	325 mg PO daily for 4–6 wk.
Unfractionated heparin	Inactivating thrombin and activated factor X (factor Xa) through an antithrombin-dependent mechanism.	5000 units SC every 8–12 h while immobilized.
Low molecular weight heparin (Enoxaparin)	Binds to antithrombin III and accelerates activity. Inhibits thrombin and factor Xa.	30 mg SC every 12 h × 7–10 d. Consider 21 d if immobile
Rivaroxaban	Selectively blocks factor Xa, inhibiting blood coagulation.	10 mg PO qd × 12 d.
Dabigatran	Directly and reversibly inhibits thrombin.	220 mg PO qd × 28 d. Start with 110 mg PO for first day.

Abbreviations: INR, international normalized ratio; PO, by mouth; qd, every day; SC, subcutaneous.

In a review by Mangwani and colleagues,[20] pharmacologic prophylaxis did not statistically reduce the risk of DVT or PE with the use of dalteparin or tinzaparin in 4 randomized studies.[27–30] In contrast, 3 other studies concluded that LMWH (reviparin, fraxiparin) reduced the incidence of DVT significantly in trauma patients.[20,31–33] A meta-analysis by Testroote and colleagues[20,34] established that administration of LMWH led to a decreased rate of DVT in lower limb trauma requiring immobilization, both with and without surgical intervention. A related retrospective study showed that there is no difference in VTE rates in foot and ankle surgery with the use of antiplatelet therapy (aspirin).[20,35] Another study found an increased incidence of DVT in higher risk patients (prior history of DVT, malignancy, oral contraceptive use, and obesity), despite having chemical prophylaxis. In addition, this patient population received prophylaxis for an average of 2.8 days and yet their risks of DVT were not diminished.[20,36] A 142-patient prospective study performed by Saragas and colleagues[37] analyzed whether chemoprophylaxis had any impact on the prevention of VTE in a cohort of foot and ankle surgical patients requiring the combination of below-knee cast immobilization and non–weight bearing for greater than or equal to 4 weeks. The patients were administered a rivaroxaban regimen postoperatively, and the primary outcome measure was clinical VTE confirmed by ultrasonography or perfusion scanning. The investigators discovered that oral pharmacologic thromboprophylaxis significantly reduces the risk of VTE in patients requiring cast immobilization and non–weight bearing following foot and ankle surgery. The risk/benefit ratio favors this treatment as opposed to the treatment of major morbidity following nonfatal VTE.[37] In a separate international double-blind, placebo-controlled study on foot and ankle fractures, Zheng and colleagues[38] reported that routine anticoagulant prophylaxis was not found to be necessary. Raphael and colleagues[39] compared the most effective agents for prophylaxis against DVT in total joint arthroplasty, after an American Academy of Orthopedic Surgeon's statement suggested the use of aspirin. The investigators found that overall symptomatic PE rate was lower ($P<.001$) in patients receiving aspirin (0.14%) than in the patients receiving warfarin (1.07%). This difference did not change after matching.

CLINICAL CONSENSUSES AND LITERATURE RECOMMENDATIONS
Prophylaxis Opponents

Mangwani and colleagues[20] weighed the overall risk for foot and ankle surgery against the overall population, and their recommendations line up with Fleischer and colleagues[21] that patients with no known risk, who are normally ambulatory, should not receive chemical prophylaxis. The investigators noted that the consensus found throughout the literature suggests that there is unclear evidence and little to no variation between the randomized controlled trials with respect to pharmacologic agents, doses, and initiation of therapy.[20,27,29,31,32] Mizel and colleagues[40] analyzed the low-dose warfarin levels on DVT and its relationship to unwarranted nonfatal PE and bleeding. They discovered that although warfarin did keep the prothrombin levels at approximately 1.5 times the normal level, it did increase the incidence of severe postoperative bleeding. Given the low incidence of DVT after foot and ankle surgery, the investigators concluded that the costs and potential complications involved are not justified for the small gain that may accrue. In a large prospective foot and ankle surgery study (n = 201), Solis and Saxby[41] found that deep calf clots were identified in just 3.5% of the population, but none of these showed extension in the proximal calf based on ultrasound and therefore did not require routine prophylaxis. Furthermore, Wukich and Waters[42] presented a 1000-patient retrospective study analyzing

VTE after forefoot, midfoot, hindfoot, and ankle procedures over the course of 1.5 years. They found that 4 had developed VTE, with 3 developing further nonfatal PE. The consensus argued against the use of routine prophylactic postoperative treatment and suggests the need for high-powered evidence studies.[42] Expanding on that, the current practice in the United Kingdom with respect to the NICE guidelines has investigators skeptical and pressing for high-powered prospective studies as suggested by Wukich and Waters.[42] The English study raises concerns that the guidelines for assessing the need for routine use of chemical prophylaxis in foot and ankle surgery does not assess outcomes for regimens without chemical intervention, considering mortality of heparin prophylaxis has been estimated at 2.5 times higher than the estimated rate of fatal PE reported in the study.[43,44] Furthermore, Griffiths and colleagues[35] explored the incidence of VTE in elective foot and ankle surgery with and without aspirin prophylaxis. The study compared 1078 patients who received 75 mg aspirin as routine thromboprophylaxis between 2003 and 2006, with 1576 patients with no form of aspirin between 2007 and 2010. The incidence rate was 0.42% (excluding those lost to follow-up) with 0.27% and 0.15% denoted DVT and PE accruals, respectively. The investigators concluded that because the incidence rate of VTE following surgery was at insignificant rates, the routine use of prophylaxis was not warranted, with the exception of high-risk groups. On the other hand, Robertson and Roche[45] reviewed the importance of prophylaxis in major amputations of the lower extremity in the UK literature and found varying suggestions. Several observational studies supported the use of thromboprophylaxis; one study reported that DVT occurred in 50% of people following major lower extremity amputation without prophylaxis. Another randomized study showed a similar 10% incidence rate of DVT in the LMWH versus unfractionated heparin groups. Still, the use of pharmacologic thromboprophylaxis (with LMWH) with concomitant VTE remains high, so the use of mechanical methods has been suggested, although obvious contraindications in an amputee is assumed. In general, the investigators found the Scottish Intercollegiate Guidelines Network had conflicting results about the overall efficacy of prophylaxis not only in the amputee community, but post foot and ankle surgery, and noted the need for extensive systematic reviews remains important.[45]

Prophylaxis Proponents

A large level I prospective, double-blinded, placebo-controlled trial was performed to evaluate the efficacy and safety of subcutaneous reviparin in patients who required immobilization in a plaster cast for at least 5 weeks after a leg fracture or rupture of the Achilles tendon. Lassen and colleagues[32] discovered that the routine use of reviparin for Achilles tendon injuries is beneficial. Likewise, Saragas and colleagues[37] analyzed an 88-patient retrospective study on the high incidence rate of DVT in Achilles tendon repair, and strongly concluded that a routine VTE prophylactic regimen be considered for patients undergoing major orthopedic surgery. In a non–weight bearing cast study, Saragas and colleagues found alarming rates of 5.09% VTE development in their hallux subgroup that contained patients not requiring immobilization and were allowed to weight bear, and an even higher value at 8.46% was found in their cast/non–weight bearing group. The investigators felt that prophylactic treatment should be administered and should continue until the patient regains adequate mobility either by weight bearing or removal of immobilization between 28 and 42 days.[46]

Prophylaxis Case by Case

In a report by Shibuya and colleagues,[47] the incidence of acute DVT and PE in foot and ankle trauma was evaluated using the National Trauma Data Bank. The investigators found that risk factors associated with acute DVT (older age, obesity, higher injury score) were statistically significant drivers, but that population was low. The investigators concluded that routine pharmacologic prophylaxis might not be indicated in foot and ankle trauma, but individual assessment of the risk factors associated with acute DVT/PE is important and therefore could not come to a uniform decision on a reasonable routine.[47] In a level II meta-analysis by Calder and colleagues,[48] 43,381 patients were evaluated for VTE and the incidence with and without chemical intervention was clinically assessed at 0.6% and 1%, respectfully. Radiologically, the values were 12.5% and 10.5%, respectfully, which provides an interesting comparison of clinical and radiological presentation of VTE and subsequent diagnosis. The investigators also noted an increased clinical incidence of 7% and radiological incidence of 35.3% in Achilles tendon repair. Not surprisingly, the investigators concluded that isolated foot and ankle surgery has a lower incidence when compared with similar lower limb VTE events. With the exception of Achilles tendon repair (which did not show differences in surgical or conservative succeeding DVT events), the routine use of chemical prophylaxis is not justified in those undergoing isolated foot and ankle surgery, but a patient-specific plan needs to be followed nonetheless.

Consensus Recommendations

Clear guidelines have not been established for VTE prophylaxis in the realm of foot and ankle surgery. The American College of Foot and Ankle Surgeons (ACFAS) has formulated a clinical consensus statement that is composed of surgical subspecialty experts who have established guidelines to manage patients in the postoperative course.[49] The reason why DVT prophylaxis has been poorly elucidated is due to the varying complexity of lower extremity procedures/injuries, as well as the differing postoperative protocols. The incidence of DVT after a diverse review of hindfoot arthrodesis, total ankle replacement, ankle fracture surgery, and first metatarsal surgery was reported to be 0.3% in database of 90,000 patients.[49] Varying reports of incidence have also been documented. For example, in separate studies using phlebography, DVT was reported as high as 28% to 36% following ankle surgery.[49]

The ACCP guidelines in 2012 had recommended pneumatic compression of the lower extremity for mechanical DVT prophylaxis and that chemical therapy is not always necessary. The guidelines did not address the ranging complexity of lower extremity procedures and was only addressing fatal or symptomatic DVT or PE. The ACFAS panel of experts sought out to answer 4 questions: (1) Is routine chemical prophylaxis warranted after foot/ankle surgery or injury requiring immobilization? (2) If routine prophylaxis is not warranted, which patients should receive chemical prophylaxis? (3) Which method(s) of VTED prophylaxis is/are preferred? (4) Which diagnostic tests should be used for an individual suspected of DVT?

After the panel reviewed the literature, each question was addressed given the evidence in the presently available database. The panel concluded that routine chemical prophylaxis is not always indicated. Within the realm of major knee and hip surgeries, the incidence of VTE was reported to be 50% or higher.[49] However, when comparing foot and ankle surgeries, the evidence showed that at 3-month and 6-month follow-ups, the incidence was 0.3%.[49] Determining which patient warrants chemical prophylaxis has much to do with the risks and benefits of each patient. According to the consensus, there are 3 broad categories: patient-specific, related to the treatment course, and related to the surgery or injury itself. Furthermore, risk factors were subdivided into 2 groups: primary and secondary risk factors. Primary risk factors include previous history of VTED, prolonged immobilization, hypercoagulable state, and previous cancer history. Secondary risk factors entail obesity, advanced age older than

60 years, oral contraceptives, family history of VTED, varicosities, severity of injury, and diabetes. After each patient is examined and the risk factors are assessed, it will guide the provider if VTED prophylaxis is necessary. Once the decision has been made, the next course of action is to decide what type of chemical prophylaxis is necessary. In a multimodal approach, there are 5 strategies that help minimize the incidence of VTE: (1) stopping oral contraceptives/hormone replacement therapy 4 weeks before surgery, (2) limiting duration of hospital stay, (3) intermittent pneumatic compression, (4) early rehabilitation and mobilization of limb, and (5) chemical prophylaxis. LMWH is an effective way to reduce incidence of VTE and seems to be favored among foot and ankle surgeons. There are reports of decreased incidence by 50% in surgical and nonsurgical patients requiring immobilization.[49] The risk was far less in nonsurgical patients when coupled with LMWH. Although the risks are low, there are potentially significant complications with LMWH that include significant prolonged bleeding and thrombocytopenia. Studies had shown occurrences of 0.26% upward to 8%.[49] The complications were mitigated by immediate discontinuation of LMWH as well as blood transfusions. Aspirin was also reviewed and noted lack of high-level evidence addressing the efficacy of this drug. Another study showed no difference in postoperative VTED comparing the group that took aspirin and the control group that did not. The consensus from ACFAS stated that patients may be better suited with warfarin maintaining an INR between 2 and 3, or other oral agents that do not require INR monitoring, such as apixaban, dabigatran, or rivaroxaban. Timing is another important issue when administering chemical prophylaxis. LMWH therapy is recommended to begin 12 to 24 hours after the surgical procedure. No added benefits were noted starting chemical prophylaxis preoperatively. The panel also agreed that chemical prophylaxis should be continued for the duration of the immobilization period. Inferior vena cava filter use was mainly reserved for patients who had history of VTED and when chemical prophylaxis was contraindicated. Their final point addressed which diagnostic test is appropriate for ruling out VTED. In large part, the decision for the diagnostic test revolves around a patient's history, which is associated with patient risk factors including the Wells criteria.[26] If there is a low probability, then a D-dimer would suffice. If the pretest risk assessment is high, especially with a high Wells score, then a venous ultrasound study may be warranted. The panel recommended that scanning of the entire leg that is symptomatic is a safe method and that bilateral serial scans are not necessary.

On review of the literature, the panel's consensus is that not every foot and ankle procedure warrants DVT prophylaxis. Each patient must undergo a risk stratification to determine the appropriate course of prevention. Diagnostic measures are also tailored to each individual patient, which will help guide the patient's treatment. When taking into consideration all risk factors, each patient will have an individualized treatment protocol in preventing postoperative VTED.

SUMMARY

The extensive literature on the decision for prophylaxis of DVT is inconclusive. Most authors are opponents for the routine prophylactic administration, citing consequential bleeding and hemorrhage in the chemical arm, and the lack of efficacy in the mechanical arm as driving factors to render routine prophylaxis as ineffective. Despite the risks, the incidence of subsequent DVT and PE remains minute, as compared with hip and knee outcomes. In an expert opinion e-mail response query by Shah and colleagues[50] regarding the current practice of DVT prophylaxis in foot and ankle surgery, they received 80 committee member responses regarding 3 scenarios: (1)

a 50-year-old woman with no risk factors, (2) a 50-year-old woman with a history of PE, and (3) a 35-year-old woman actively using birth control pills. The responses correlate with the overwhelming literature synopsis to oppose routine prophylaxis, while continuing to support the overall insecurity of physicians to implement such ideology into accepted common practice. The data showed 57% of respondents believe "no prophylaxis is required" for scenario 1, 97.5% believe "yes prophylaxis required" for scenario 2, and 49% believe "some prophylaxis is required" for scenario 3. The wide variation is of no surprise based on the current standard of care for patients with or without potential for the subsequent development of VTE following foot and ankle surgery. Park and colleagues[51] recently made substantial strides to audit a large sum of records using the VTE risk assessment tool (RAT) to assist in screening of in-patients at a single hospital over a 2-year span who received thromboprophylaxis. Their standardized VTE RAT model increased thromboprophylaxis usage and decreased PE rates, with an even greater improvement for their surgical arm population. They highlighted the necessity and utter importance of a multidimensional, standardized model to combating VTE. Foot and ankle surgeons need to continue to stay vigilant and educated through audits, prescribing tools, and electronic reminder systems. Even at an insignificant frequency rate, a lower extremity postsurgical prophylaxis model to be implemented and validated remains a top priority. It is the hope of the authors of this article that future research will be devoted to high-powered prospective studies to verify and authenticate a stratification prototype that will change and improve the standard of care for the lower extremity community.

REFERENCES

1. Malay DS. Venous thromboembolism associated with foot and ankle surgery. Complications in foot and ankle surgery. Springer; 2017. p. 9–27.

2. Pengo V, Lensing AW, Prins MH, et al. Incidence of chronic thromboembolic pulmonary hypertension after pulmonary embolism. N Engl J Med 2004;350(22): 2257–64.

3. Schade VL, Roukis TS. Antithrombotic pharmacologic prophylaxis use during conservative and surgical management of foot and ankle disorders: a systematic review. Clin Podiatr Med Surg 2011;28(3):571–88.

4. Slaybaugh RS, Beasley BD, Massa EG. Deep venous thrombosis risk assessment, incidence, and prophylaxis in foot and ankle surgery. Clin Podiatr Med Surg 2003;20(2):269–89.

5. Esmon CT. Basic mechanisms and pathogenesis of venous thrombosis. Blood Rev 2009;23(5):225–9.

6. Rosendaal FR. Venous thrombosis: a multicausal disease. Lancet 1999; 353(9159):1167–73.

7. Esmon CT, Schwarz HP. An update on clinical and basic aspects of the protein C anticoagulant pathway. Trends Cardiovasc Med 1995;5(4):141–8.

8. Schwarz HP, Fischer M, Hopmeier P, et al. Plasma protein S deficiency in familial thrombotic disease. Blood 1984;64(6):1297–300.

9. Kunz G, Ireland HA, Stubbs PJ, et al. Identification and characterization of a thrombomodulin gene mutation coding for an elongated protein with reduced expression in a kindred with myocardial infarction. Blood 2000;95(2):569–76.

10. Biguzzi E, Merati G, Liaw PC, et al. A 23bp insertion in the endothelial protein C receptor (EPCR) gene impairs EPCR function. Thromb Haemost 2001;86(04): 945–8.

11. Sevitt S. The structure and growth of valve-pocket thrombi in femoral veins. J Clin Pathol 1974;27(7):517–28.

12. Paterson J, Mclachlin J. Precipitating factors in venous thrombosis. Surg Gynecol Obstet 1954;98(1):96–102.

13. Lund F, Diener L, Ericsson JL. Postmortem intraosseous phlebography as an aid in studies of venous thromboembolism: with application on a geriatric clientele. Angiology 1969;20(3):155–76.

14. Bovill EG, van der Vliet A. Venous valvular stasis-associated hypoxia and thrombosis: what is the link? Annu Rev Physiol 2011;73:527–45.

15. Saha P, Humphries J, Modarai B, et al. Leukocytes and the natural history of deep vein thrombosis: current concepts and future directions. Arterioscler Thromb Vasc Biol 2011;31(3):506–12.

16. Esmon CT, Owen WG. Identification of an endothelial cell cofactor for thrombin-catalyzed activation of protein C. Proc Natl Acad Sci U S A 1981;78(4):2249–52.

17. Esmon CT. The roles of protein C and thrombomodulin in the regulation of blood coagulation. J Biol Chem 1989;264(9):4743–6.

18. Kostadima E, Zakynthinos E. Pulmonary embolism: pathophysiology, diagnosis, treatment. Hellenic J Cardiol 2007;48(2):94–107.

19. Goldhaber SZ, Elliott CG. Acute pulmonary embolism: part I: epidemiology, pathophysiology, and diagnosis. Circulation 2003;108(22):2726–9.

20. Mangwani J, Sheikh N, Cichero M, et al. What is the evidence for chemical thromboprophylaxis in foot and ankle surgery? Systematic review of the English literature. Foot (Edinb) 2015;25(3):173–8.

21. Fleischer AE, Abicht BP, Baker JR, et al. American College of Foot and Ankle Surgeons' clinical consensus statement: risk, prevention, and diagnosis of venous thromboembolism disease in foot and ankle surgery and injuries requiring immobilization. J Foot Ankle Surg 2015;54(3):497–507.

22. Amaragiri SV, Lees T. Elastic compression stockings for prevention of deep vein thrombosis. Cochrane Database Syst Rev 2000;(3):CD001484.

23. Urbankova J, Quiroz R, Kucher N, et al. Intermittent pneumatic compression and deep vein thrombosis prevention. A meta-analysis in postoperative patients. Thromb Haemost 2005;94(6):1181.

24. Sachdeva A, Dalton M, Amaragiri SV, et al. Elastic compression stockings for prevention of deep vein thrombosis. Cochrane Database Syst Rev 2010;(7):CD001484.

25. Delaney JA, Opatrny L, Brophy JM, et al. Drug–drug interactions between antithrombotic medications and the risk of gastrointestinal bleeding. Can Med Assoc J 2007;177(4):347–51.

26. Scarvelis D, Wells PS. Diagnosis and treatment of deep-vein thrombosis. Can Med Assoc J 2006;175(9):1087–92.

27. Goel D, Buckley R, Devries G, et al. Prophylaxis of deep-vein thrombosis in fractures below the knee: a prospective randomised controlled trial. J Bone Jt Surg Br 2009;91(3):388–94.

28. Lapidus LJ, Ponzer S, Elvin A, et al. Prolonged thromboprophylaxis with Dalteparin during immobilization after ankle fracture surgery: a randomized placebo-controlled, double-blind study. Acta Orthop 2007;78(4):528–35.

29. Lapidus LJ, Rosfors S, Ponzer S, et al. Prolonged thromboprophylaxis with dalteparin after surgical treatment of Achilles tendon rupture: a randomized, placebo-controlled study. J Orthop Trauma 2007;21(1):52–7.

30. Jørgensen PS, Warming T, Hansen K, et al. Low molecular weight heparin (Inno-hep) as thromboprophylaxis in outpatients with a plaster cast: a venografic controlled study. Thromb Res 2002;105(6):477–80.

31. Kujath P, Spannagel U, Habscheid W. Incidence and prophylaxis of deep venous thrombosis in outpatients with injury of the lower limb. Haemostasis 1993; 23(Suppl. 1):20–6.

32. Lassen MR, Borris LC, Nakov RL. Use of the low-molecular-weight heparin revi-parin to prevent deep-vein thrombosis after leg injury requiring immobilization. N Engl J Med 2002;347(10):726–30.

33. Kock H, Schmit-Neuerburg K, Hanke J, et al. Thromboprophylaxis with low-molecular-weight heparin in outpatients with plaster-cast immobilisation of the leg. Lancet 1995;346(8973):459–61.

34. Testroote M, Stigter W, de Visser DC, et al. Low molecular weight heparin for pre-vention of venous thromboembolism in patients with lower-leg immobilization. Co-chrane Database Syst Rev 2008;(4):CD006681.

35. Griffiths J, Matthews L, Pearce C, et al. Incidence of venous thromboembolism in elective foot and ankle surgery with and without aspirin prophylaxis. J Bone Jt Surg Br 2012;94(2):210–4.

36. Hanslow SS, Grujic L, Slater HK, et al. Thromboembolic disease after foot and ankle surgery. Foot Ankle Int 2006;27(9):693–5.

37. Saragas NP, Ferrao PN, Jacobson BF, et al. The benefit of pharmacological venous thromboprophylaxis in foot and ankle surgery. S Afr Med J 2017;107(4): 327–30.

38. Zheng X, Li DY, Wangyang Y, et al. Effect of chemical thromboprophylaxis on the rate of venous thromboembolism after treatment of foot and ankle fractures. Foot Ankle Int 2016;37(11):1218–24.

39. Raphael IJ, Tischler EH, Huang R, et al. Aspirin: an alternative for pulmonary em-bolism prophylaxis after arthroplasty? Clin Orthop Relat Res 2014;472(2):482–8.

40. Mizel MS, Temple HT, Michelson JD, et al. Thromboembolism after foot and ankle surgery. Clin Orthop 1998;348:180–5.

41. Solis G, Saxby T. Incidence of DVT following surgery of the foot and ankle. Foot Ankle Int 2002;23(5):411–4.

42. Wukich DK, Waters DH. Thromboembolism following foot and ankle surgery: a case series and literature review. J Foot Ankle Surg 2008;47(3):243–9.

43. Hamilton P, Hariharan K, Robinson A. Thromboprophylaxis in elective foot and ankle patients—current practice in the United Kingdom. Foot Ankle Surg 2011; 17(2):89–93.

44. Jameson SS, Augustine A, James P, et al. Venous thromboembolic events following foot and ankle surgery in the English National Health Service. J Bone Jt Surg Br 2011;93(4):490–7.

45. Robertson L, Roche A. Primary prophylaxis for venous thromboembolism in peo-ple undergoing major amputation of the lower extremity. Cochrane Database Syst Rev 2013;(12):CD010525.

46. Saragas NP, Ferrao PNF, Saragas E, et al. The impact of risk assessment on the implementation of venous thromboembolism prophylaxis in foot and ankle sur-gery. Foot Ankle Surg 2014;20(2):85–9.

47. Shibuya N, Frost CH, Campbell JD, et al. Incidence of acute deep vein throm-bosis and pulmonary embolism in foot and ankle trauma: analysis of the National Trauma Data Bank. J Foot Ankle Surg 2012;51(1):63–8.

48. Calder JD, Freeman R, Domeij-Arverud E, et al. Meta-analysis and suggested guidelines for prevention of venous thromboembolism (VTE) in foot and ankle surgery. Knee Surg Sports Traumatol Arthrosc 2016;24(4):1409–20.
49. Meyr AJ, Mirmiran R, Naldo J, et al. American College of Foot and Ankle Surgeons((R)) clinical consensus statement: perioperative management. J Foot Ankle Surg 2017;56(2):336–56.
50. Shah K, Thevendran G, Younger A, et al. Deep-vein thrombosis prophylaxis in foot and ankle surgery: what is the current state of practice? Foot Ankle Spec 2015;8(2):101–6.
51. Park MY, Fletcher JP, Hoffmann C, et al. Prevention of venous thromboembolism through the implementation of a risk assessment tool: a comparative study in medical and surgical patients. Int Angiol 2018. [Epub ahead of print].

Prevention of Infection in Foot and Ankle Surgery

John Boyd, DPM*, Richard Chmielewski, MD

KEYWORDS

- Prophylactic antibiotics • Infection prevention • Surgical site infection
- Patient comorbidities • Skin preparation and risk stratification

KEY POINTS

- Prophylactic antibiotics, although important, are only a part of an infection prevention strategy.
- Appropriate risk stratification involves patient-related, surgeon-related, and procedure related factors.
- Obtaining a detailed patient history and physical provides practitioners with invaluable patient-related information that is important to infection risk stratification.
- Specific machinations related to surgery performed in the preoperative, operative, and postoperative time frames must be optimized to limit infection.
- Appropriate postoperative management aids in reducing postoperative wound complications and surgical site–related infection.

INTRODUCTION

In 2014, 17.2 million hospital visits involved invasive, therapeutic surgeries, with bunionectomy and digital surgeries accounting for 1.6% (272,000).[1] Foot and ankle surgery is far from immune to the exponential advances seen across all surgical specialties. Scope of practice continues to broaden and, as it does, the amount and complexity of surgery performed increase as well. Podiatric surgery is a unique field in which a variety of pathology is treated on a routine basis, ranging from implant-related orthopedics to removal of soft tissue masses to diabetic foot infections to open fractures on any given operative day. This process encompasses the entire spectrum of operative wounds based on contamination, exposing the surgeon to different infectious risks on a case-by-case basis[2] (**Table 1**). Postoperative infections after foot and ankle surgery are reported as high as 6.5%[3] and, anatomically, the lower

Disclosure Statements: None.
Section of Podiatry, Department of Surgery, St. Vincent Charity Medical Center, 2322 East 22nd Street, Cleveland, OH 44115, USA
* Corresponding author.
E-mail address: JohnBoydDPM@gmail.com

Clin Podiatr Med Surg 36 (2019) 37–58
https://doi.org/10.1016/j.cpm.2018.08.007
0891-8422/19/© 2018 Elsevier Inc. All rights reserved.

Table 1
Classification of surgical procedures by degree of contamination and risk of subsequent infection

Type of Procedure	Definition	Wound Infection Rate (%) Preoperative Antibiotics Administered	
		No	Yes
Clean	Atraumatic; no break in technique; gastrointestinal, genitourinary, and respiratory tracts not entered	5.1	0.8
Clean-contaminated	Gastrointestinal or respiratory tract entered but without spillage; oropharynx, sterile genitourinary, or biliary tract entered; minor break in technique	10.1	1.3
Contaminated	Acute inflammation; infected bile or urine; gross spillage from gastrointestinal tract	21.9	10.2
Dirty	Established infection	40	10

From Measley RE. Antimicrobial prophylaxis: prevention of postoperative infection [Chapter 3]. In: Merli GJ, Weitz HW, editors. Medical management of the surgical patient. Philadelphia: Elsevier; 2008. p. 37; with permission.

extremity, specifically the foot and ankle, may be at a greater risk for the development of these infections.[4,5] In 2010, Berkes and colleagues[4] reported on a review of all acute (within 6 weeks of initial surgery) postoperative infections at 3 level 1 trauma centers over a 2-calendar-year period (2004 and 2005). In total, 123 infections in 121 patients met inclusion criteria for analysis. Anatomic frequency of the 123 infections were as follows: (1) upper extremity—15/123 (12%); (2) pelvis—18/123 (18%); (3) femur—19/123 (19%); and (4) tibia/fibula/ankle/foot—63/123 (51%).

Because of this prevalence and the significant morbidity, cost, and even mortality associated with postoperative infections, the podiatric surgeon must be acutely aware of risk factors that may predispose to this unwanted result from surgical intervention. In this article, postoperative infections are referred to as surgical site infections (SSIs). SSIs occur within 30 days of surgery or within 90 days of surgery if prosthetic material is implanted[6] and are divided into superficial incisional (skin and subcutaneous tissue), deep incisional (deep fascia, tendon, and muscle), and organ/space (bone and osteoarticular).[7] Potentially significant ramifications can be experienced by the patient, surgeon, and health care facility due to SSIs.[7–9] For further details, see https://www.halyardhealth.com/media/1515/patient_risk_factors_best_practices_ssi.pdf. A comprehensive plan to prevent postoperative infections should be fashioned and used for each surgical candidate.

RISK STRATIFICATION

Much of the risk stratification is based on factors inherently attributed to the patient, surgeon, and/or procedure. From a temporal standpoint, the process of evaluating these factors from an infectious perspective and implementing appropriate measures of prevention are sorted into 3 different time frames: preoperative, operative, and postoperative. All 3 periods are essential in the understanding of the development of an infection and the hopeful prevention and/or appropriate treatment thereof. These time frames are not mutually exclusive. The information obtained and preventive steps taken in the preoperative phase undoubtedly has an effect on operative prevention and postoperative assessment and plan of action for SSIs.

PREOPERATIVE PHASE

The preoperative phase of risk stratification begins with assessment of the patient via a standard history and physical. Pertinent patient risk factors for SSIs may be related to medical comorbidities, abnormal physical findings, and/or pharmacologics (prescribed or not) and commonly include the following: diabetes, renal disease, liver disease, substance abuse, peripheral neuropathy, tobacco use, obesity, low preoperative serum albumin, malnutrition, concurrent steroid use, prolonged preoperative stay, poor integument quality, remote infection at the time of surgery, presence of retained hardware from previous orthopedic surgery, and colonization with *Staphylococcus aureus*.[3,10,11] These factors are either modifiable or not modifiable. As an example, age and the presence of retained hardware are factors in which modification cannot be achieved. Some factors, such as the presence of a remote infection, are modifiable, and appropriate actions should be taken, whereas other factors, such as glycemic control in a diabetic, obesity, and nutrition, are only modifiable to a certain extent. Any factor in which improvement can be reasonably attained, however, should be achieved or at the very least attempted. It cannot be overemphasized how valuable the involvement of other specialists can be to optimize patients for surgery and to re-emphasize to patients the importance of this optimization.

Identification of patient-related factors allows for a more plausible and accurate discussion of the surgery with the patient in regard to risk of infection and success of procedure. The presence of significant risk(s) may argue against having a certain procedure because the patient and the surgeon may ascertain that the attendant risks outweigh perceived benefits of a proposed surgery. This kind of patient education and patient involvement in decision making improves the entire surgical process from a patient's vantage point and provides realistic expectations.[11]

One of the strongest considerations for postponing an elective foot and ankle surgery is the presence of a remote infection. The classic example is a patient who presents the day of surgery with a suppurative paronychia. The paronychia should be treated and resolved prior to performing elective orthopedic type foot and ankle surgery. With the renaissance and escalation of ankle implant arthroplasty in the recent past, other remote infections, such as urinary tract infections (UTIs) and periodontal disease, are more concerning because these infections often are asymptomatic and unnoticed until the day of surgery. In these 2 instances, transient bacteremia can be produced with oral manipulation during intubation or with bladder catheterization perioperatively. In a retrospective case-controlled study, Kouvoularis and colleagues[12] identified 58 total joint arthroplasties (total hip replacements and total knee replacements) in which a wound infection developed out of a total of 19,735 surgeries, for an infection rate of 0.29%. Of the 58 wound infections, there were concomitant 7 UTIs (3 preoperative and 4 postoperative), all of which were treated. The offending pathogen with respect to wound infections was nonenteric 80% of the time and in only 1 instance did the wound pathogen match the UTI pathogen. The authors concluded that treated UTIs presented a very low risk as an origin for a surgically related wound infection. Active UTIs should be treated and, if bacteremia is suspected from an oral or urinary source, appropriate antibiotic coverage for the source of the bacteremia should be instituted.[10]

The presence of a remote infection at the time of surgery represents an unnecessary and potentially correctable risk. Valentine and colleagues[13] review 2349 clean surgical wounds for a minimum of 38 months after procedures. Preoperatively, there was a documented remote infection in 208/2349 cases or 8.9% of the time prior to surgery. In these instances of remote infection, antibiotics were either given therapeutically, started prior to 24 hours before surgery, or as a standard prophylactic antibiotic. A postoperative infection was documented in a total of 178 patients: 30 of these infections were seen in the 208 cases of a remote infection identified preoperatively (30/208 — 14.4%) whereas only 148 postoperative infections were seen in the remaining patients, which did not demonstrate a remote infection preoperatively (148/2141 — 6.9%). The postoperative infection rate was double in patients with a remote infection preoperatively. Also, the patients with a remote infection and given therapeutic antibiotics experienced infection one-third of the time compared with the same class of patients just given prophylactic antibiotics. Another investigator has reported remote infections increase the probability of an SSI by a factor of 3 to 5.[9] As an example, in an urgent case, such as an unstable ankle fracture where a remote skin infection has been identified on the preoperative surgical visit, it is prudent to introduce empiric antibiotics therapy for suspected infecting organisms prior to surgery and potentially consult infectious disease, depending on the severity of the remote infection and the immune status of the patient.

Inflammatory skin manifestations, such as eczema and dermatitis, have been shown to predispose toward an SSI.[14,15] Appropriate dermatology consultation and resolution of the skin problem are recommended prior to an elective surgery.[10,11] Again, in the instance of an urgent surgery, appropriate antibiotic coverage for

Staphylococcus species is warranted. The need to identify potential remote infections highlights the importance of a thorough review of systems at a patient's preoperative surgical visit. Simply asking questions, such as, "Have you had a recent infection for which you took an antibiotic?" or "Do you have a history of infections?" goes a long way toward identifying remote infections and potentially avoiding an unnecessary complication. Also, make sure to get a copy of current medications from the patient's pharmacy, because often patients are on an antibiotic and either do not know that they are on the antibiotic or do not know why they are on the antibiotic. This is not uncommon in elderly patients.

Age has been long debated as to whether it is a direct, independent factor for increasing the probability of a postoperative infection. The debate centers on the question, Is it increased age that causes increased incidence of postoperative infections or is the higher prevalence of comorbid conditions making age an indirect factor? This is an important question due to the fact that by 2020, patients over the age of 65 will become the largest segment of the surgical patient demographic.[16] Another important factor to consider with age is that other problems that are associated with aging also increase the probability of postoperative complications, including infection. These include the following: cognitive impairment, frailty, immobility/functional capacity, poor nutrition, and postoperative discharge/transitional difficulties.[17] Again, these issues are more common experiences in the elderly—age greater than 65—but any or all of these items can be seen in patients less than 65. In a multi-institutional, retrospective study of 144,485 consecutive surgical patients with 1684 postoperative SSIs (rate 1.2%), Kaye and colleagues[18] investigated the relationship of age and its effect on risk of postoperative SSIs. Statistical analysis demonstrated a direct relationship with age and an increased risk of SSI seen as an increased risk of 1.1% per year of age from the ages of 17 to 65. In patients aged 65 years or older, there was an inverse relationship between age and risk of SSI with the risk of SSI decreasing 1.2% for each year. An explanation given by the investigators for this decrease of SSI after 65 was a selective bias may have existed where surgeons would not operate on older patients (due to an increase in comorbidities seen in this group of patients) to decrease the likelihood of postoperative complications.[18] In a recent retrospective analysis of 1510 ankle fractures from 3 institutions, however, Sun and colleagues[19] demonstrated infection rates in the 3 following age groups: (1) age less than 50: 902/926 (97.4%) without SSI and 24/926 (2.6%) with SSI; (2) age 50 to 69: 503/538 (93.5%) without SSI and 35/538 (6.5%) with SSI; and (3) age greater than 69: 35/42 (83%) without SSI and 7/42 (16.7%) with SSI. Their conclusion was that increasing age was a direct and independent variable related to establishment of an SSI.

Other comorbidities that are potentially modifiable, such as obesity, diabetes, malnutrition, nicotine consumption, and specific medications, should be recognized and addressed via primary care physician or specialists. This type of intervention reduces the chances of infection in these instances and, again, demands that patients have an active role in the preparation for their surgery.

Obesity, defined as a body mass index (BMI) greater than 30 kg/m^2, is the second leading cause of death in the United States[20] and accounts for the expenditure of a significant amount of health care dollars, well over $200 billion annually.[21,22] This topic resonates with many foot and ankle specialists because obesity comprises a significant percentage of patients with lower extremity complaints, specifically common pathologies of the foot and ankle. Obesity is potentially modifiable. However this is time consuming irrespective of method: Surgery with lifestyle modifications versus isolated lifestyle modifications. Although obesity is associated with other comorbidities, such as diabetes, metabolic syndrome, and cardiac disease, an elevated BMI has been shown a significant risk factor for the development of postoperative complications, specifically infection.[22] A proposed mechanism for increased infection postulates that obesity adversely affects the immune status of the patient. Decreased peripheral tissue oxygenation is another proposed mechanism for increased infections in obese patients.[23,24] It has been demonstrated that obese patients have decreased subcutaneous oxygen tension in both open[23] and laparoscopic[24] abdominal surgeries.

In a retrospective evaluation of postoperative complications within 30 days in 7271 patients after moderate or major noncardiac surgery, analysis was performed to evaluate complication parameters in obese versus nonobese patients. An overall complication rate of 7.7% (7,271/94,853) was observed and there were statistically significant discrepancies between obese and nonobese patients in regard to myocardial infarction, peripheral nerve injury, wound infection, and UTI. Specifically, wound infections were appreciated in 3.5% (237/6773) of the nonobese patients and in 6.0% (133/2217) of the obese patients. The same difference was seen regarding both superficial and deep infections.[25]

Dowsey and Choong[26] retrospectively analyzed prospectively collected date in 1207 consecutive cases of primary hip arthroplasty. Patients were divided into 4 groups with respect to BMI: normal (<25 kg/m^2), overweight (25–29 kg/m^2), obese (30–39 kg/m^2), and morbidly obese (>39 kg/m^2). A significantly higher rate of deep infection was reported in the obese and morbidly obese patient groups and this association was independent and did not correlate with comorbidities such a diabetes, cardiovascular disease, operative time, transfusion requirements, the use of a drain, or cement requirements. In another study, the same investigators prospectively looked at 1214 consecutive primary total knee replacements and found 18 infections within the first year postoperatively for an infection rate of 1.5%: "There were no prosthetic infections in diabetic patients who were not obese."[27]

Another modifiable risk factor that has become more and more prevalent is diabetes.[28] Although there are questions as to whether diabetes is an independent risk factor for infection after surgery and at what level (Hb)A$_{1c}$ represents a tipping point to avoid elective surgery,[29] there is a clear association between poorly controlled diabetes and a generalized increase in perioperative morbidity, specifically SSI. In 1 study, general surgery patients with a preoperative glucose level greater than 220 mg/dL had an infection rate 2.7 times that of general patients with a glucose level below 220 mg/dL.[30] A 1.59 relative risk increase of postoperative infection for every 1% increase in HbA$_{1c}$ above 7.0% is seen after foot and ankle surgery.[31] Postoperative glucose levels over 200 mg/dL during the first 48 hours are associated with increased risk of SSI.[32,33] While striving to optimize the preoperative HbA$_{1c}$, it is evident in some cases that targeted levels may not be obtainable.[34] In purely elective situations, this may preclude the patient from having the surgery. In instances where surgery is a necessity to allow for stable ambulation, however, an interactive discussion should take place with patient in regard to the increase in risk for the development of an infection. More importantly, in all diabetic patients, discussion of preoperative glucose control is an opportunity to impress on these patients the merits of glucose control. In many instances, these discussions concerning a particular surgery may represent a life-lasting change that precipitates the improvement of other facets of the diabetes and ultimately improve the quality and duration of a patient's life.

Malnutrition represents another potentially modifiable risk factor that can have significant impact on a patient's ability to heal and the development of an SSI.[7] Malnutrition is usually diagnosed via abnormal laboratory markers, abnormal anthropometric measurements, and standardized assessments.[35] Anthropometric measurements typically involve calf circumference, arm muscle circumference, and triceps skin fold whereas the more common laboratory criterion are albumin (<3.5 g/dL), serum transferrin (<200 mg/dL), and total lymphocyte count (<1500 mm^3).[35] Malnutrition mechanism for an increase in SSI results from an impairment in wound healing[36] due to diminished fibroblast proliferation and collagen synthesis,[37] an exaggeration in inflammation,[38] and impairment of the immune system secondary to lymphocytopenia.[37] The most commonly used parameter for diagnosing malnutrition in the orthopedic literature is the serum albumin level[37,39] and, based on laboratory values alone, the most common definition of malnutrition in orthopedics is a deficiency in at least 1 of common laboratory values (albumin, transferrin, and lymphocyte count) [cross].[35] Yi and colleagues[40] looked at the association of laboratory parameters indicating malnutrition and a potential independent link to the occurrence of an acute periarticular joint infection after a revisional procedure. A retrospective review of 501 lower extremity joint revisions (126 septic and 375 aseptic etiologies) by the same surgeon over a 9-year period revealed that malnutrition was an independent marker for a periarticular infection in both patients with septic and aseptic causes for joint revision.[40] A retrospective analysis was performed on prospectively collected data by the American College of Surgeons National Surgical Quality Improvement Program, which is a prospective surgical registry. This initially comprised a total of 101,523 total hip and knee arthroplasty patients for the purpose of evaluating hypoalbuminemia and its effect on specific postoperative complications experienced within 30 days of surgery. Exclusionary criteria, presence of preoperative serum albumin levels, produced a final study population of 49,603 of 101,523 (48.9%). Of the 49,603 studied individuals, 1,964 (4.0%) had low preoperative albumin levels. Nine different complications had an occurrence rate of greater than 0.1%, and each was compared separately to the existence of hypoalbuminemia. All complications presented at a significantly higher rate, before and after statistical adjustment, when serum albumin level was less than 3.5 g/dL. The most notable outlier was the frequency of SSI, where there was a 2-fold increase in patients with hypoalbuminemia. A low albumin level was a meaningful, independent risk factor for pneumonia and SSI.[37]

In many instances, malnutrition is potentially modifiable and, once recognized, should be evaluated for etiology and possible intervention. Consideration for dietary consultation from nutritional specialist, dental consultation, swallowing study, medication review by primary care physician, family intervention, and social service evaluation should be contemplated in this group of patients. Obvious reasons, such as poverty, lack of access to nutrition, and age-related impairments, may not be apparent on initial evaluation of patient. In the elderly patient population, issues, such as reduced appetite, presence of numerous chronic disease processes, multiple medication requirements, history of depression, and decreased metabolism, are commonly connected to the cause of malnutrition. Perioperatively, it is important to control the amount of time these patients are fasting. As with most complex medical problems, a multispecialty solution is usually the most effective and expedient pathway.

Predilection toward a postoperative infection can be seen in patients exposed to ongoing glucocorticoid therapy, especially for treatment of chronic disease. There is an incidence of increased SSIs in patients with Crohn disease receiving ongoing steroid treatment prior to abdominal surgery.[41,42] In a neurosurgery study of 26,634 patients, preoperative steroid use was found an independent risk factor for the development of postoperative infections.[43] Appropriate consultation with the prescribing physician and an infectious disease specialist should be sought to determine reducing or eliminating steroids alone or in conjunction with a patient-specific tailored antibiotic regimen.

Smoking tobacco and nicotine use contributes to poor health and decreases life expectancy in general and has been shown to significantly increased morbidity and mortality in patients undergoing surgery.[44] Specific to surgical outcomes, nicotine use is an independent risk factor for SSI because it delays primary wound healing. This is, in part, due to microvasculature constriction and microcirculation congestion due to platelet aggregation[45] and nonfunctioning hemoglobin.[46,47] Many articles have shown an increase in wound complications and infection after surgery in patients who smoke versus nonsmokers.[48–51] Sørensen[52] performed a meta-analysis to investigate postoperative infection and wound complications in smokers, former smokers, and nonsmokers. When comparing smokers and nonsmokers in 140 cohort studies, the adjusted odd ratio was 3.6 for necrosis, 2.07 for delayed healing and dehiscence, 1.79 for SSI, and 2.27 for wound complications. Four randomized controlled trials specifically looked at the effect of smoking cessation. Only wound infection, out of all healing complications, was statistically reduced.[52]

In some patients, cessation of smoking is not possible due to the urgency of the required procedure, ie, open reduction and internal fixation ankle fracture; however, in patients undergoing many elective surgeries, intervention is potentially warranted and feasible. In these instances, the patient should be referred to the primary care physician or a smoking cessation program of repute. Some health care providers mandate documentation of nicotine abstinence before elective surgery can be scheduled and/or completed.

Skin carriage, surveillance, and decolonization of *Staphylococcus* species present a complex and controversial topic, but there must be recognition and a plan of action for patients who are at increased risk for developing *Staphylococcus* species SSIs from an endogenous source (patient). Approximately 20% of healthy patients are persistent carriers (same strain for extended periods of time) and 30% are intermittent carriers (different strains over time)[53] and the most common anatomic location for carriage is the anterior nares.[54] Overwhelmingly, the most common organism for postoperative infections, especially in orthopedic surgery, is *Staphylococcus aureus*. Transitively, there is a positive association between skin carriage of *Staphylococcus aureus* species and the development of an SSI, and multiple meta-analyses endorsed the relationship between the presence of *Staphylococcus* species in the nares and the development of SSIs. In patients who have had positive nasal cultures and developed an SSI, the organism responsible for the SSI matched the organism from nasal cultures up to 85% of the time.[55]

Despite this information, there is hesitance to adopt a universal surveillance and culture-directed decolonization program.[10] The reticence is based on the quality of literature done to this point because there are few, if any, level 1 studies completed in this area of research. Methodology and inferior numbers of many studies cause concern when contemplating the adoption of widespread surveillance and decolonization.[56–59] Also, there is a question of cost benefit[10] even though, intuitively, it would seem the cost saved by infections prevented would far outweigh the cost of implementing a universal surveillance program. There is a need for better method of design with respect to investigation into this problem. New recommendations from the Infectious Diseases Society of America on this topic are due to be published in 2019. Irrespective of the scientific deficiencies, many institutions, especially with respect to total knee and hip arthroplasty, routinely surveil for skin carriage of *Staphylococcus* species.

In the interim, the most prudent course of action argues to approach this on a case-by-case basis.[10,56,57] In patients who have a prior history of staphylococcus species infections, prior SSI, or history of skin conditions susceptible to

Staphylococcus infections; in sufficiently immunocompromised patients; and in patients undergoing significant surgery with concerning medical comorbidities,[10,56,57] preoperative surveillance and decolonization are recommended and implementation should be based on specific institutional protocol. In situations where surgery is urgent (results of surveillance cultures not available) and there is a high risk for skin carriage, such as previous methicillin-resistant *Staphylococcus aureus* (MRSA) infection, empiric use of nasal mupirocin should be considered.

PERIOPERATIVE/OPERATIVE PHASE

This section focuses on separate components of the surgical process. Specific characteristics inherent to a specific surgery may represent the most important risk factors that predispose a particular procedure and patient to an infection. The following 4 characteristics can have influence on the inception of a postoperative infection: (1) abdominal surgical procedure; (2) procedure lasting greater than 2 hours; (3) contaminated, dirty, or infected procedure by traditional classification; and (4) 3 or more discharge diagnoses that increase the complexity of a patient's condition.[60] Of these 4 characteristics, 3 of them occur in foot and ankle surgery on a relatively frequent basis. Classically, an increase risk for SSI in a particular surgery was attributed to length over 2 hours, American Society of Anesthesiologists classification greater than 2, and surgical contamination class of contaminated or infected.[61] In a systematic review (328 publications truncated to 57 inclusions) of risk factors associated with SSIs, Korol and colleagues[62] identified reduced patient fitness and increased hospital exposure time, patient frailty, surgery duration, and complexity as emblematic for SSIs. Because a time limit of 2 hours is somewhat arbitrary, Culver and colleagues[63] recommended a system designed to be able to compare surgeons of like and different disciplines to each other. This is based on the time it takes to perform a particular surgery and how this time compares with the 75th percentile generated among a registry of surgeons. Above or below the 75th percentile designates whether the procedure is protracted in nature, and this 75th percentile time differs as the level of acuity of a particular surgery is elevated, that is, coronary artery bypass grafting has a higher level of acuity compared with cholecystectomy.[61,63] Several investigators cite an increased surgical time as a concern for a subsequent SSI.[64–67] An increased time between incision and closure raises time of contamination irrespective of category or complexity of any procedure. In a systematic review of 81 studies concerning operative time as a risk for an SSI, Cheng[65] noted that patients with an SSI had an operative time of at least 30 minutes greater than patients without an SSI across all procedure types and surgical disciplines. After adjusting for numerous patient and operative risks, Proctor[68] demonstrated that the duration of a surgery was an independent risk factor when reviewing multiple general surgery procedures in the American College of Surgeons National Surgical Quality Improvement Program data base. As an example, in cases of isolated laparoscopic cholecystectomy, infectious complications were 1.4% in cases lasting 1.1 hours to 1.5 hours compared with a rate of 0.7% in cases less than or equal to 0.5 hours.

At the time of surgery, there are antimicrobial and nonantimicrobial interventions that can be instituted to minimize infection. Most attention has been focused on prophylactic antibiotics as the most integral part of the operative experience with regard to avoiding an infection. Many elements outside of prophylactic antibiotics, however, such as appropriate skin preparation, judicious Electrocautery use, and limited room traffic, can have a profound effect on decreasing SSIs.

Prophylactic Antibiotics

At the outset, many health care facilities and institutions mandate antibiotic prophylaxis in all surgeries and the ensuing discussion may be just an exercise in academics, but the information is important. The argument for compulsory, preoperative antibiotics stems largely out of fear of not preventing an infection. As an example, Measley[2] cites infection rates with and without preoperative antibiotics in all 4 wound classifications, from clean through dirty. Rates are as follows: (1) clean—0.8% and 5.1%; (2) clean-contaminated—1.3% and 10.1%; (3) contaminated—10.2% and 21.9%; and (4) dirty—10% and 40%, with and without antibiotics, respectively, for all 4 classes.[1] Concerns for giving prophylactic antibiotics in every elective surgical procedure are driven, however, by potential untoward, inflammatory or other drug reactions, anaphylaxis, cost, and the perpetuation of drug resistance organisms.

The literature relating to antibiotic prophylaxis for elective foot surgery is incomplete at best and practice habits in regard to this topic have emanated largely from orthopedic investigations and other multidisciplinary panels. Dayton and DeVries,[56] in a systematic review of the literature, identified only 6 principal articles directly investigating perioperative prophylactic antibiotics in clean elective foot surgery.[5,69–73] Consensus statements from Dayton and DeVries[56] were largely adopted from other sources due to small numbers in and methodology of foot literature.[6,74–83] Again, recommendations as to whether an antibiotic should be used in a prophylactic fashion revolve around procedure-related and patient-related factors. Antibiotics are recommended for elective foot procedures in patients with significant comorbidities, patients taking medications that predispose to infection, and patients who are inherently immunocompromised. These patient parameters are irrespective of type and/or length of procedure. Procedures where antibiotics are recommended involve bone, implants/hardware, and increased length of procedure; however, length of procedure is often not clarified. With respect to soft tissue procedures, there is no clear recommendation and the decision is a surgeon preference. As an example, in a simple ganglion excision overlying the distal extensor hallucis longus tendon involving a healthy patient, antibiotics may not be necessary, whereas a surgery involving an extensive dissection for the removal of a multiloculated giant cell tumor from the anterior ankle should merit consideration for the use of preoperative antibiotics.[6,56]

Antibiotics should be narrow in spectrum and directed at the most likely pathogen— *Staphylococcus aureus*. Cefazolin is ideal for surgical prophylaxis in orthopedic type surgery due to coverage of normal skin flora, low risk of immediate hypersensitivity reactions, low cost, and bioavailability. Cefazolin is the drug of choice for clean foot and ankle procedures and is dosed at 2 g for patients under 120 kg and 3 g for patients at or above 120 kg. In patients with β-lactam allergies, clindamycin or vancomycin is recommended. Dosing for clindamycin is 900 mg and for vancomycin is 15 mg/kg in patients with normal kidney function. Clindamycin is used more and more often due to limited drug reactions and no kidney issues compared with vancomycin and a desire to preserve the efficacy of vancomycin. Vancomycin should be given over at least an hour to avoid red man syndrome–associated infusion of this medication in less than an hour.

In the absence of a β-lactam allergy, routine prophylactic utilization of vancomycin for any procedure is currently not recommended.[6] On a case-by-case basis, prophylactic vancomycin may be considered. As an example, in cases of recent hospitalization or a nursing home patient, vancomycin should be considered an appropriate choice for prophylaxis due to increased prevalence of MRSA in this patient subgroup. Vancomycin is inferior to cefazolin in regard to methicillin-sensitive *Staphylococcus aureus*, and some investigators suggest giving both antibiotics as prophylaxis in these high-risk patients.[84,85]

In instances of lengthy procedures, approximately 2 half-lives of a drug should be completed before redosing the medication. As an example, the half-life of cefazolin is 1.2 hours to 2.2 hours and recommended time of redosing this prophylactic antibiotic is 4 hours. Half-lives of clindamycin and vancomycin are 4 hours to 8 hours and 2 hours to 4 hours, respectively; would rarely is ever redosed during a foot and ankle procedure and recommendation for redosing clindamycin is 6 hours.[6] A prophylactic antibiotic is typically a 1-time dose for outpatient surgery and should be discontinued at 24 hours for inpatients irrespective of indwelling catheters or drains.[6]

In the past, antibiotics were given as an "on-call to the operating room" or "at induction of anesthesia" medication, which provided marked variability as to when the antibiotic was given or if it was given at all. The American Society of Health-System Pharmacists (2013) recommends that prophylactic antibiotics should be started within 60 minutes of the incision. Medications with longer infusion times (vancomycin and fluoroquinolones) are recommended to be started within 120 minutes of skin incision.[6] In a recent retrospective review of 1933 procedures in 1632 patients over a 3.5-year time frame, Tantigate and colleagues[86] investigated whether infusion of prophylactic antibiotics less than 15 minutes prior to surgery (tourniquet inflation) represented a difference in regard to SSIs compared with infusion time of 15 minutes to 60 minutes prior to surgery. It is not uncommon for patients to receive prophylactic antibiotics just prior to skin incision. In this review, there were no differences in SSIs or wound complications between 2 groups. After stepwise multivariate logistic regression analysis, more than 90% of risk related to the development of an SSI was due to the patient's American Society of Anesthesiologists score and length of surgery.

Skin Preparation

The following nonantimicrobial items are discussed separately because they represent different and important avenues to assist in the limitation of SSIs: skin preparation, Bovie use, room traffic, and dead space management. Skin preparation does not just reference cleaning the foot just prior to the incision. Skin preparation refers to both the patient and surgeon and, in the case of the patient, applies to 2 different time frames—days before the surgery and the day of the surgery. With respect to the surgeon, traditionally water-based solutions of chlorhexidine or povidone-iodine have been used; however, alcohol-based rubs containing ethanol, isopropanol, or n-propanol are just as effective[87] and the reduction of colony-forming units on the hands of surgeons is better facilitated with alcohol rubs than chlorhexidine gluconate and povidone-iodine.[88] Current recommendations for skin preparation of surgeons' hands or operating room personnel hands, which are grossly contaminated, are to wash hands with soap and water followed by cleaning underneath nails with nail pick and then drying with paper towel. This is followed by an alcohol-based rub for 3 minutes, which is used prior to any following cases that same day. The AORN guidelines recommend a scrub brush for 3 minutes in place of the alcohol rub for the first case of the day.[89] Scrubbing in-between each case on a day in which multiple surgeries are performed can actually make the possibility of SSI worse by aggravating and increasing the skin flora of the surgeon. Good nail hygiene and cleaning out underneath fingernails decrease bacterial load prior to initial scrub. With respect to longer cases, Hosseini and colleagues[90] demonstrated that there were increased colony-forming units under gloved hands as cases progressed in time, and hand recolonization occurred at the 5-hour mark, absolutely recommending to redo surgeon skin preparation at 5 hours. Although there is no reason a surgeon cannot rescrub sooner, it seems that 5 hours is the cutoff at which this process should take place.

Proper surgical attire assists in the reduction of microbial shed from operating room personnel. This is probably most important with respect to surgeons because they have sustained contact with operative wounds. Surgical attire items are often neglected and may have contribution in the evolution of SSIs. Frequently, a surgeon uses the same surgical mask for the entire day, sometimes wearing the same mask for several cases. Zhiqing and colleagues[91] investigated surgical masks as a potential source of bacterial contamination during operative procedures. The following conclusions were made: (1) bacterial counts on the outer surface of the surgical masks were elevated with increasing surgical times; (2) when evaluating masks from the same surgeons, a marked increase in bacterial load was noted in the 2-hour group; (3) the body surface of the surgeon rather than the operating room environment was the source for bacterial contamination of the surgical mask; and (4) surgeons should change their surgical masks after each surgery, especially if greater than 2 hours.

With respect to the patient, many institutions have recommended chlorhexidine bathing prior to surgery. Currently, however, there is little evidence to support this practice and authorities now recommend bathing with soap and water for standard orthopedic surgery.[10,11,92] Although seemingly trivial, it is important for patients to use clean towels and clean linens after bathing, especially if a patient is known to have prior history of Staphylococcus infection or skin problem.[89] Hair removal should be done with a clipper the day of surgery because shaving can cause microabrasions that can increases chances of infection. Another method of reducing bacterial counts, specifically of the forefoot, is to have patient soak the foot in an antiseptic agent just prior to surgery. Ng and Adeyemo[93] compared soaking with chlorhexidine gluconate for 10 minutes to not soaking. There was a statistically significant reduction in bacteria when comparing the group who soaked (chlorhexidine) with the control group who did not soak. Because this study was performed on inpatients, potential consideration should be given to a soaking protocol because this inpatient group usually has a significant increase and perhaps alteration in skin flora due to exposure to the hospital bacterial milieu.

The recommendation for the reduction, and hopeful removal, of commensal and transient skin organisms is heralded by many organizations,[89,94–98] and the techniques used for completion of this task essentially relies on 2 variables: the antiseptic and the method of application. In general, chlorhexidine is superior to povidone-iodine skin preparation and has been shown to decrease bacterial load more effectively.[98–101] Bristles for scrub are preferred to sponges[102] and an alcohol-based preparation is optimal irrespective of chlorhexidine gluconate or povidone-iodine.[3]

Unlike most other anatomic areas, the foot represents a unique area when contemplating skin preparation techniques prior to surgery. The skin of the foot may contain up to 3 million microorganisms/cm^2.[98] The foot provides a particular setting for the presence and growth of bacteria due to paucity or absence of pilosebaceous units and apocrine sweat glands in conjunction with closed digital confinement via socks and most shoe gear.[103,104] SSIs are more common with orthopedic surgery of the foot and ankle compared with the remainder of the body.[5,105] Specifically, the forefoot, interdigital areas, and skin nail folds present a challenge with respect to skin preparation and reduction of bacteria. Proper cleansing remains difficult because of anatomic barrier of nail, hyponychium, and nail fold. Studies investigating skin antisepsis in foot and ankle surgery focus on the nail fold and interdigital areas because these 2 areas represent a nexus for persistent skin carriage of microbacteria and may be why SSIs are more frequent after foot and ankle surgery compared with other orthopedic procedures.[101,102,106] Ostrander and colleagues[107] looked at residual bacterial counts prospectively in 50 consecutive patients after 2 different skin preparation techniques: (1) 1-step povidone-iodine gel and (2) 2-step iodophor scrub followed by povidone-iodine paint. Three anatomic areas were cultures after skin preparation and draping: (1) the hallux nail fold; (2) 2/3 and 4/5 interdigital areas; and (2) anterior ankle (control). In group 1, positive cultures were seen in 76% of halluces, 68% of interdigital areas, and 16% of the controls, whereas, in group 2, there were positive cultures in 84% of halluces, 76% of interdigital areas, and 28% of the controls. The most commonly cultured organism was staphylococcus epidermidis.

Interdigital areas and hallux nail folds harbor bacteria and these areas tend to be difficult to adequately sterilize. Although it is critical to provide the best technique for skin preparation, some simple precautions may go a long way toward preventing an infection. If the surgery does not involve the forefoot, a sterile glove, Coban wrap, or Ioban drape should be fashioned to enclose the forefoot. This limits handling of the digits, nail folds, and interdigital areas. It is easy to unknowingly drag a suture through the interdigital areas when closing wounds, especially when performing forefoot surgery. When suturing wound of the forefoot, it is important to make sure the tail of the suture is away from the digits to help avoid exposing the wound to bacteria of the hallux nail fold or an interdigital area.

Both iodine and chlorhexidine are effective agents for skin antisepsis; however, with respect to foot and ankle surgery, Bibbo and colleagues[106] recommended chlorhexidine scrub with alcohol paint as preferable to a povidone-iodine scrub and paint. In a prospective, randomized controlled study, Bibbo and colleagues[106] looked at 127 patients, 67 patients in group 1 (povidone-iodine) and 60 patients in group 2 (chlorhexidine/alcohol). All patients had prophylactic antibiotics and a timed, 7-minute scrub and paint with 1 of the 2 studied antiseptic agents followed by appropriate drying and subsequent toe cultures (digits, nail folds, and all web spaces) and site of proposed surgical incision. Group 1 had a total of 53 positive cultures—5 were from proposed incisions and the remainder were positive "toe" cultures. Results from group 2 were a total of 23 positive cultures, 2 from proposed incisional areas and 21 from "toe" cultures. Group 2, the chlorhexidine/alcohol group, had significantly fewer positive cultures, group 2—23/60 (38%) versus group 1—53/67 (79%). Given that SSIs are more common in elective foot and ankle surgical patients, the investigators recommended using chlorhexidine gluconate scrub followed by alcohol paint as skin preparation agents to maximize reduction of risk for SSI.

In a simulated skin preparation study, Keblish[102] compared 4 different preparation techniques to answer the following 3 questions: (1) Does the use of an alcohol prewash provide additional efficacy to standard orthopedic povidone-iodine scrub-and-paint skin preparation? (2) Is there any difference between the efficacies of povidone-iodine vs alcohol alone? and (3) Does the use of bristles to scrub the skin provide added benefit to using sponges? There was no improvement with an added alcohol prewash to the povidone-iodine preparation. The alcohol alone preparation was superior to the povidone-iodine alone technique. The best preparation technique was alcohol scrub and paint using bristles instead of sponges for the scrub. The mechanical removal of bacteria was facilitated with the use of bristles. This study performed qualitative and quantitative culture results of the hallux nail fold, interdigital areas, and anterior ankle (control). There was a statistically significant reduction of heavy growth at the nail fold culture site in both instances where the bristle technique was used. The best skin preparation technique in this study was alcohol scrub and paint using mechanical bristle application.[102]

It is important to educate the operating room personnel as to the idiosyncrasies of skin flora, greater potential for SSIs, and differing optimal skin preparations and applications in foot and ankle surgery as opposed to standard orthopedic skin preparation prior to surgery. Although seemingly inconsequential, there are some meaningful differences that should be addressed.

Electrocautery Use

Kumagai and colleagues[108] performed a study on laboratory rats, testing strength of incisions made with either electrocautery or scalpel, and found that tensile strength was significantly less when the incision was made with electrocautery. Bacteremia was more frequent in the electrocautery group, which also had a higher mortality at 7 days. Soballe and colleagues[109] performed a similar study on laboratory rats, performing midline incisions with either cold knife, electrocautery cutting current, or electrocautery coagulation current. Incisions were also inoculated with bacterial organisms—equal parts Escherichia coli, Pseudomonas aeruginosa, Streptococcus pyogenes, and S aureus and normal saline as a control. All animals that expired postoperatively, either by complication or sacrifice, had a 2-cm^2 full-thickness tissue square excised and fixed to be histologically examined for inflammation and abscess formation. Electrocautery produced more tissue necrosis and inflammation than cold knife at all levels of bacterial inoculation, with coagulation current causing more than cutting current. Electrocautery coagulation current produced more abscesses than either electrocautery cutting current or scalpel with inoculations at 10^3 and 10^5 and produced the only abscesses seen in the wounds inoculated with only sterile saline.[109]

More recently, Prakash and colleagues[110] performed a double-blind controlled trial comparing 90 patients randomized into either scalpel or electrocautery for midline abdominal incision. Although there was an increased rate of infection in the emergency cases, they found no significant difference in infection between the electrocautery and scalpel group (14.63% vs 12.19%). Even though the Prakash and colleagues[110] study did not reveal a statistically significant difference in infection rates with use of electrocautery and scalpel, it is inherently intuitive that the use of electrocautery for the purposes of dissection should be limited because this practice increases necrotic tissue within the surgical field.[110]

Operating Room Environment

Several elements, such as laminar airflow, ultraviolet light, room traffic, and exhaust suits, comprise the operating room environment and contribute to airborne bacterial contamination. Of these items, room traffic and positive pressure in the operating room are the most pertinent topics with respect to foot and ankle surgery. Positive room pressure, which means there is elevated pressure in the operating room compared with adjacent hallways and rooms, assists in limiting the entrance of airborne contaminants into the operating room. Room sterility can also be affected by an increase in room traffic,[111] which can cause an increase in bacterial counts within the operating room.[112,113] Significant activity within the operating room causes increased room traffic and multiple entrance and exits from the operating room, which allows for loss of positive room pressure. This activity not only decreases the sterility of the operating room but also creates an environment where there is loss of focus on the job at hand. This is a relatively benign process that often occurs without notice from staff or the surgeon.

Mears[114] retrospectively evaluated 191 total knee and hip arthroplasty procedures to evaluate number and amount of time for door opening for a given case and if this would affect positive room pressure. A sensor was placed on the operating room door that recorded the number and how long the door was open during a case. Basic surgery information was recorded (surgeon name, patient name, date of surgery, and so forth) and this was matched with the door opening information and information from the heating, ventilation, and air conditioning systems. This was all done unbeknown to the surgeons and operating room staff. In 77 of the 191 cases, doors were opened for a length of time that allowed for the reversal of positive room pressure. The minimum pressure in the room was statistically affected, but the average room pressure was not; thus, the loss of positive room pressure was temporary. Doors were open a total of 8.5% of total operative time, which equaled 9.5 minutes per case. There was only 1 infection, which was not an outlier with respect to total time door was opened.

Babkin[111] reviewed total joint arthroplasties and found that there was an increase rate of infection with respect to the left lower extremity, which was closest to the operating room door. After this discovery, once the case started the operating room door was permanently shut for the remainder of a given case. The disproportionate number of infections with respect to the left side was corrected. With respect to affecting staff behaviors in regard to door opening in the operating room, Hamilton and colleagues[115] showed that simply monitoring the door had no effect on the reduction of door openings, but door openings decreased significantly after a mandatory seminar on the importance of door openings and the reduction of SSIs.

Another issue to consider is the order in which cases are done. Technically, once a room is turned over it should be clean; however, it is prudent to complete purely elective cases at the beginning of the operative day and schedule infections at the end. Many institutions have rooms in which only total joints are performed. This is something to consider in specific foot and ankle cases, such as total ankle implant arthroplasty and osteochondral grafts.

Dead Space Management

In every surgical discipline, adequate hemostasis is a cornerstone of good surgical practice. Invariably, there are certain procedures in which hemostasis is difficult. In foot and ankle surgery, cases such as calcaneal fractures, Charcot reconstruction and virtually any revisional hindfoot or ankle case present challenges with respect to bleeding. The use of a drain in these instances helps manage dead space and persistent bleeding and potentially prevent a postoperative complication or infection by avoiding or limiting a hematoma. In instances when a drain is not used, either a hematoma forms or blood extravasation causes a macerated wound, which can lead to wound healing problems and or infection. A Jones compression dressing is almost always used in a cases where a drain is implemented. The combination of a compression dressing and a drain minimizes the possibility of hematoma formation and subsequent wound problems. It is important to monitor output of the drain and to remove the drain in an appropriate time frame, typically by the first dressing change at the latest. Leaving the drain in too long can increase the risk of infection.[116]

POSTOPERATIVE

Postoperatively, there a few items that must be addressed to avoid a postoperative infection. First, all exit and entrance points to the body via lines and catheters should be minimized or eliminated as soon as feasible. Drains and Foley catheters should be discontinued as soon as possible to minimize any transient bacteremia and remove any point of external continuity to the operative wound. Other forms of infection or potential infection, such as atelectasis or pneumonia, should be preemptively reduced in occurrence rate by instituting incentive spirometry, respiratory therapy, and mobilization via physical therapy. Arrangements for this same type of approach should be made preoperatively for patients who have procedures done on an outpatient basis. Demonstration and instructions on incentive spirometry can and should be done preoperatively for the outpatient procedures as well as physical therapy to maximize safe and protected mobility at home after surgery.

In general, the original postoperative dressing should stay intact for at least 24 hours to 48 hours. The dressing should remain clean, dry, and intact. Dressings that are blood soaked should not be reinforced because allowing the persistence of moisture at the wound edge increases the bacterial count and cause wound maceration, which often progresses to a dehiscence, a wound complication with or without infection. If dressing is blood soaked 24 hours postoperatively, a sterile dressing change should be performed with reapplication of a compression dressing. This is not infrequently seen in cases, such as status post repair of a calcaneal fracture. This area of the foot is intolerant to less than optimal wound conditions.

SUMMARY

Traditionally, infection prevention has largely focused on prophylactic antibiosis. Over the past 25 years, a process has evolved to incorporate inherent risks related to the patient, procedure, and surgeon into a risk-stratification process to identify and potentially prevent SSIs in high-risk situations. It is incumbent on the surgeon to engage in this process and inform the patient as to the risk-to-benefit ratio of desired results of a given procedure and the attendant risks of the same. Patient involvement and education portend improved patient satisfaction almost irrespective of procedure results or adverse outcomes. In these instances, this process and the communication thereof assist in the mitigation of untoward outcomes and help preserve the patient-doctor relationship. Also, the appropriate involvement of other specialists preoperatively and postoperatively cannot be overemphasized. This routine confers confidence to patient in regard to a particular course of action and underscores the importance of identified risk factors and potential or realized complications.

REFERENCES

1. Steiner CA, Karaca Z, Moore BJ, et al. Surgeries in hospital-based ambulatory surgery and hospital inpatient settings, 2014 Healthcare Cost and Utilization Project. Rockville (MD): Agency for Healthcare Research and Quality (US); 2006. Available at: https://www.ncbi.nlm.nih.gov/pubmed/28722845.
2. Measley RE. Antimicrobial prophylaxis: prevention of postoperative infection [Chapter 3]. In: Merli GJ, Weitz HW, editors. Medical management of the surgical patient. Philadelphia: Elsevier; 2008. p. 35–50.
3. Butterworth M, Payne T. Surgical infections [Chapter 5]. In: Lee MS, Grossman JP, editors. Complications in foot and ankle surgery: management strategies. New York: Springer; 2017. p. 69–87.
4. Berkes M, Obremskey WT, Scannell B, et al. Maintenance of hardware after postoperative infection following fracture internal fixation. J Bone Joint Surg Am 2010;92:823–8.
5. Miller WA. Postoperative wound infection in foot and ankle surgery. Foot Ankle Int 1983;4:102–4.
6. Bratzler DW, Dellinger EP, Olsen KM, et al, American Society of Health-System Pharmacists (ASHP), Infectious Diseases Society of America (IDSA), Surgical Infection Society (SIS), Society for Healthcare Epidemiology of America

(SHEA). Clinical practice guidelines for antimicrobial prophylaxis in surgery. Surg Infect (Larchmt) 2013;14(1):73–156.

7. Pear SM. Patient risk factors and best practices for surgical site infection prevention. Halyard Health - Managing infection control; 2007. p. 56–64.

8. Kirkland KB, Briggs JP, Trivette SL, et al. The impact of surgical-site infections in the 1990s: attributable mortality, excess length of hospitalization, and extra costs. Infect Control Hosp Epidemiol 1999;20(11):725–30.

9. Edwards LD. The epidemiology of 2056 remote site infections and 1966 surgical wound infections occurring in 1865 patients: a four year study of 40,923 operations at Rush-Presbyterian-St. Luke's Hospital, Chicago. Ann Surg 1976;184(6): 758–66.

10. Miller AO, Brause BD. Infection and perioperative orthopedic care [Chapter 22]. In: Mackenzie CR, Cornell CN, Memtsoudis SG, editors. Perioperative care of the orthopedic patient. New York: Springer; 2014. p. 259–65.

11. Bosco JA, Slover JD, Haas JP. Perioperative strategies for decreasing infection. a comprehensive evidence-based approach. J Bone Joint Surg Am 2010;92: 232–9.

12. Kouvoularis P, Sculco P, Finerty E, et al. Relationship between perioperative urinary tract and infection and deep infection after joint arthroplasty. Clin Orthop Relat Res 2009;467(7):1859–67.

13. Valentine JR, Weigelt JA, Dryer D, et al. Effect of remote infections on clean wound infection rates. Am J Infect Control 1986;14(2):64–7.

14. Boguniewicz M, Leung DY. Atopic dermatitis: a disease of altered skin barrier and immune dysregulation. Immunol Rev 2011;242(1):233–46.

15. Lim CT, Tan KJ, Ang KC. Implant infection caused by dermatitis: a report of two cases. J Orthop Surg (Hong Kong) 2007;15(3):365–7.

16. Etzioni DA, Liu JH, Maffart MA, et al. The aging population and its impact on the surgery workforce. Ann Surg 2003;238(2):170–7.

17. MacKenzie CR, Cornell CN. Perioperative care of the elderly orthopaedic patient [Chapter 18]. In: Mackenzie CR, Cornell CN, Memtsoudis SG, editors. Perioperative care of the orthopedic patient. New York: Springer; 2014. p. 209–19.

18. Kaye KS, Schmit K, Pieper C, et al. The effect of increasing age on the risk of surgical site infection. J Infect Dis 2005;191:1056–62.

19. Sun Y, Wang H, Tang Y. Incidence and risk factors for surgical site infection after open reduction internal fixation of ankle fracture. A retrospective multicenter study. Medicine (Baltimore) 2018;97(7):1–6.

20. Mokdad AH, Marks JS, Stroup DF, et al. Actual causes of death in the United States, 2000. JAMA 2004;291:1238–45.

21. Bookman JS, Schwarzkopf R, Rathod P, et al. Obesity: the modifiable risk factor in total joint arthroplasty. Orthop Clin North Am 2018;49:291–6.

22. Stewart M. Obesity in elective foot and ankle surgery. Orthop Clin North Am 2018;49:371–9.

23. Kabon B, Nagele A, Reddy D, et al. Obesity decreases perioperative tissue oxygenation. Anesthesiology 2004;100:274–80.

24. Fleischmann E, Kurz A, Niedermayr M, et al. Tissue oxygenation in obese and non-obese patients during laparoscopy. Obes Surg 2005;15:813–9.

25. Bamgbade OA, Rutter TW, Nafiu OO, et al. Postoperative complications in obese and nonobese patients. World J Surg 2007;31:556–60.

26. Dowsey MM, Choong PF. Obesity is a major risk factor for prosthetic infection after primary hip arthoplasty. Clin Orthop Relat Res 2008;466:153–8.

27. Dowsey MM, Choong PF. Obese diabetic patients are at a substantial risk for deep infection after primary total knee arthroplasty. Clin Orthop Relat Res 2009;467:1577–81.

28. Guyer AJ. Foot and ankle surgery in the diabetic population. Orthop Clin North Am 2018;49:381–7.

29. Lopez LF, Reaven PD, Harman SM. Review: the relationship of HbA1c to postoperative surgical risk with an emphasis on joint replacement surgery. J Diabetes Complications 2017;31:1710–8.

30. Furlong K, Ahmed I, Jabbour S. Perioperative management of endocrine disorders [Chapter 12]. In: Merli GJ, Weitz HW, editors. Medical management of the surgical patient. Philadelphia: Elsevier; 2008. p. 411–52.

31. Humpfers JM, Shibuya N, Fluhman BL, et al. The impact of glycosylated hemoglobin on wound-healing complications and infection after foot and ankle surgery. J Am Podiatr Med Assoc 2014;104(4):370–9.

32. Zerr KJ, Furnary AP, Grunkemeier GL, et al. Glucose control lowers the risk of wound infection in diabetics after open heart operations. Ann Thorac Surg 1997;63(2):356–61.

33. Terranova A. The effects of diabetes mellitus on wound healing. Plast Surg Nurs 1991;11(1):20–5.

34. Giori NJ, Ellerbe LS, Bowe T, et al. Many diabetic total joint arthroplasty candidates are unable to achieve a preoperative hemoglobin A1c of 7% or less. J Bone Joint Surg Am 2014;96:500–4.

35. Cross MB, Yi PH, Thomas CF, et al. Evaluation of malnutrition in orthopaedic surgery. J Am Acad Orthop Surg 2014;22:193–9.

36. Guo JJ, Yang H, Qian H, et al. The effects of different nutritional measurements on delayed wound healing after hip fracture in the elderly. J Surg Res 2010; 159(1):503–8.

37. Bohl DD, Shen MR, Kayupov E, et al. Hypoalbuminemia Independently predicts surgical site infection, pneumonia, length of stay, and readmission after total joint arthroplasty. J Arthroplasty 2016;31:15–21.

38. Seibert DJ. Pathophysiology of surgical site infection in total hip arthroplasty. Am J Infect Control 1999;27(6):536–42.

39. Alfargieny R, Boldalal Z, Bendardaf R, et al. Nutritional status as a predictive marker for surgical site infection in total joint arthroplasty. Avicenna J Med 2015;5(4):117–22.

40. Yi PH, Frame RM, Vann E, et al. Is potential malnutrition associated with septic failure and acute infection after revision total joint arthroplasty? Clin Orthop Relat Res 2015;473:175–82.

41. Post S, Betzler M, vonDitfurth B, et al. Risks of intestinal anastomoses in Crohn's disease. Ann Surg 1991;213(1):37–42.

42. Nguyen GC, Elnahas A, Jackson TD. The impact of preoperative steroid use on short-term outcomes following surgery for inflammatory bowel disease. J Crohns Colitis 2014;8:1661–7.

43. Merkler AE, Saini V, Kamel H, et al. Preoperative steroid use and the risk of infectious complications after Neurosurgery. Neurohospitalist 2014;4(2):80–5.

44. Turan A, Mascha EJ, Roberman D, et al. Smoking and perioperative outcomes. Anesthesiology 2011;114(4):837–46.

45. Jones JK, Triplett RG. The relationship of cigarette smoking to impaired intraoral wound healing: a review of evidence and implications for patient care. J Oral Maxillofac Surg 1992;50(3):237–9 [discussion: 239–40].

46. Hussey LC, Leeper B, Hynan LS. Development of the sternal wound infection prediction scale [review] [44 refs]. Heart Lung 1998;27(5):326–36.
47. Hotter A. The physiology and clinical implications of wound healing. Plast Surg Nurs 1984;4:4–13.
48. Lind J, Kramhøft M, Bødtker S. The influence of smoking on complications after primary amputations of the lower extremity. Clin Orthop Relat Res 1991; 267(267):211–7.
49. Veeravagu A, Patil CG, Lad SP, et al. Risk factors for postoperative spinal wound infections after spinal decompression and fusion surgeries. Spine 2009;34(17): 1869–72.
50. Lotfi CJ, Cavalcanti Rde C, Costa e Silva AM, et al. Risk factors for surgical-site infections in head and neck cancer surgery. Otolaryngol Head Neck Surg 2008; 138(1):74–80.
51. Fang A, Hu SS, Endres N, et al. Risk factors for infection after spinal surgery. Spine 2005;30(12):1460–5.
52. Sørensen LT. Wound healing and infection in surgery. The clinical impact of smoking and smoking cessation: a systematic review and meta-analysis. Arch Surg 2012;147(4):373–83.
53. Wertheim HF, Melles DC, Vos MC, et al. The role of nasal carriage in Staphylococcus aureus infections. Lancet Infect Dis 2005;5:751–62.
54. QueY, Moreillon P. Staphylococcus aureus (including Staphylococcal toxic shock syndrome) [Chapter 196]. In: Bennett JE, Dolin R, Blaser MJ, editors. Principles and practice of infectious disease. 8th edition. Philadelphia: Elsevier; 2015. p. 2237–71.
55. Weiser MC, Moucha CS. The current state of screening and decolonization for the prevention of Staphylococcus aureus surgical site infection after total hip and knee arthroplasty. J Bone Joint Surg Am 2015;97:1449–58.
56. Dayton P, DeVries JG. American college of foot and ankle surgeons' clinical consensus statement: perioperative prophylactic antibiotic use in clean elective foot surgery. J Foot Ankle Surg 2015;54(2):273–9.
57. Levy PY, Ollivier M, Drancourt M, et al. Relation between nasal carriage of Staphylococcus aureus and surgical site infection in orthopedic surgery: the role of nasal contamination. A systematic literature review and meta-analysis. Orthop Traumatol Surg Res 2013;99:645–51.
58. Price CS, Williams A, Philips G, et al. Staphylococcus aureusnasal colonization in preoperative orthopaedic outpatients. Clin Orthop Relat Res 2008;446: 2842–7.
59. Schweizer M, Perencevich E, McDaniel J, et al. Effectiveness of a bundled intervention of decolonization and prophylaxis to prevent gram positive surgical site infections after cardiac and orthopedic surgery: systematic review and meta-analysis. BMJ 2013;346:f2743.
60. Haley RW, Culver DH, Morgan WM, et al. Identifying patients at high risk of surgical wound infections: a simple multivariate index of patient susceptibility and wound contamination. Am J Epidemiol 1985;121:206–15.
61. Gaynes R, Edwards JR. National nosocomial infections surveillance system: overview of nosocomial infections caused by gram-negative bacilli. Clin Infect Dis 2005;41:848–54.
62. Korol E, Johnston K, Waser N, et al. A systematic review of risk factors associated with surgical site infections among surgical patients. PLoS One 2013;8(12): e83743.

63. Culver DH, Horan TC, Gaynes RP, et al. Surgical wound infection rates by wound class operative procedure, and patient risk index. Am J Med 1991;91: 152S–7S.
64. Leong G, Wilson J, Charlett A. Duration of operation as a risk factor for surgical site infection: comparison of English and US data. J Hosp Infect 2006;63(3): 255–62.
65. Cheng H, Chen BP, Soleas IM, et al. Prolonged operative duration increases risk of surgical site infections: a systematic review. Surg Infect (Larchmt) 2017;18(6): 722–35.
66. Peersman G, Laskin R, Davis J. Prolonged operative time correlates with increased infection rate after total knee arthroplasty. HSS J 2006;2(1):70–2.
67. Isik O, Kaya E, Dundar HZ, et al. Surgical site infection: re-assessment of the risk factors. Chirurgia (Bucur) 2015;110(5):457–61.
68. Procter LD, Davenport DL, Bernard AC. General surgical operative duration is associated with increased risk-adjusted infectious complication rates and length of hospital stay. J Am Coll Surg 2010;210(1):60–5.e1-2.
69. Zgonis T, Jolly GP, Garbalosa JC. The efficacy of prophylactic intravenous antibiotics in elective foot and ankle surgery. J Foot Ankle Surg 2004;43:97–103.
70. Paiement GD, Renaud E, Dagenais G, et al. Double-blind randomized prospective study of the efficacy of antibiotic prophylaxis for open reduction and internal fixation of closed ankle fractures. J Orthop Trauma 1994;8:64–6.
71. Reyes C, Barnauskas S, Hetherington V. Retrospective assessment of antibiotic and tourniquet use in an ambulatory surgery center. J Foot Ankle Surg 1997;36: 55–62.
72. Akinyoola AL, Adegbehingbe OO, Odunsi A. Timing of antibiotic prophylaxis in foot and surgery. J Foot Ankle Surg 2011;50:374–6.
73. Deacon JS, Wertheimer SJ, Washington JA. Antibiotic prophylaxis and tourniquet application in podiatric surgery. J Foot Ankle Surg 1996;35:344–9.
74. Boxma H, Broekhuizen T, Patka P, et al. Randomized controlled trial of single dose antibiotic prophylaxis used in surgical treatment of closed fractures: the Dutch trauma trial. Lancet 1996;347(9009):1133–7.
75. Gillespie WJ, Walenkamp GH. Antibiotic prophylaxis for surgery for proximal femoral and other closed long bone fractures. Cochrane Database Syst Rev 2010;(3):CD000244.
76. AlBuhairan B, Hind D, Hutchinson A. Antibiotic prophylaxis for wound infections in total joint arthroplasty: a systematic review. J Bone Joint Surg Br 2008;90: 915–9.
77. Formaini N, Jacob P, Willis L, et al. Evaluating the use of preoperative antibiotics in pediatric orthopedic surgery. J Pediatr Orthop 2012;32:732–5.
78. Tosti R, Fowler J, Dwyer J, et al. Is antibiotic prophylaxis necessary in elective soft tissue hand surgery? Orthopedics 2012;35:e829–33.
79. W-Dahl A, Toksvig-Larsen S. Infection prophylaxis: a prospective study in 106 patients operated on by tibial osteotomy using the hemicallotasis technique. Arch Orthop Trauma Surg 2006;126:441–7.
80. Bratzler DW, Houck PM. Antimicrobial prophylaxis for surgery: an advisory statement from the national surgical infection prevention project. Clin Infect Dis 2004;38:1706–14.
81. Dobzyniak MA, Fischgrund JS, Hankins S, et al. Single versus multiple does antibiotic prophylaxis in lumbar disc surgery. Spine 2003;28:e453–5.

82. Fonseca SNS, Kunzle SRM, Junqueira MJ, et al. Implementing 1-dose antibiotic prophylaxis for prevention of surgical site infection. Arch Surg 2006;141: 1109–13.

83. Lovato C, Wagner JD. Infections rates following perioperative prophylactic antibiotic versus postoperative extended regimen prophylactic antibiotics in surgical management of mandibular fractures. J Oral Maxillofac Surg 2009;67: 827–32.

84. Finkelstein R, Rabino G, Mashiah T, et al. Vancomycin versus cefazolin prophylaxis for cardiac surgery in the setting of a high prevalence of methicillin-resistant staphylococcal infections. J Thorac Cardiovasc Surg 2002;123: 326–32.

85. Bull AL, Worth LJ, Richards MJ. Impact of vancomycin surgical prophylaxis on the development of methicillin sensitive Staphylococcus aureus surgical site infections: report from Australian surveillance data (VICNISS). Ann Surg 2012; 256(6):1089–92.

86. Tantigate D, Jang e, Seetharaman M, et al. Timing of antibiotic prophylaxis for preventing surgical site infections in foot and ankle surgery. Foot Ankle Int 2017;38(3):283–8.

87. Parienti JJ, Thibon P, Heller R, et al, Antisepsie Chirurgicale des Mains Study Group. Hand rubbing with an aqueous alcoholic solution vs. traditional surgical hand-scrubbing and 30-day surgical site infection rates. JAMA 2002;288:722–7.

88. Hajipour L, Longstaff L, Cleeve V, et al. Hand washing rituals intrauma theatre: clean or dirty? Ann R Coll Surg Engl 2006;88:13–5.

89. AORN. Guideline for preoperative patient skin antisepsis. AORN guidelines for perioperative practice. Denver (CO): AORN, Inc.; 2016. p. 41–64.

90. Hosseini P, Mundis GM Jr, Eastlasck R, et al. Do longer surgical procedures result in greater contamination of surgeon's hands? Clin Orthop Relat Res 2016;474(7):1707–13.

91. Zhiqing L, Yongyun C, Wenxiang C, et al. Surgical masks as source of bacterial contamination during operative procedures. J Orthop Translat 2018;14:57–62.

92. Webster J, Osborne S. Preoperative bathing or showering with skin antiseptics to prevent surgical site infection. Cochrane Database Syst Rev 2007;(2):CD004985.

93. Ng AB, Adeyemo FO. Preoperative footbaths reduce bacterial colonization of the foot. Foot Ankle Int 2009;30(9):860–4.

94. Mangram AJ, Horan TC, Pearson ML, et al. Guideline for prevention of surgical site infection, 1999. Hospital Infection Control Practices Advisory Committee. Infect Control Hosp Epidemiol 1999;20:250–78 [quiz: 279–80].

95. Allegranzi B, Bischoff P, de Jonge S, et al. WHO guidelines development group new who recommendations on preoperative measures for surgical site infection prevention: an evidence based global perspective. Lancet Infect Dis 2016;16: 276–87.

96. Allegranzi B, Zayed B, Bischoff P, et al, WHO Guidelines Development Group. New WHO recommendations on intraoperative and postoperative measures for surgical site infection prevention: an evidence-based global perspective. Lancet Infect Dis 2016;16:288–303.

97. Association for Perioperative Practice. Standards and recommendations for safe perioperative practice. Harrogate (North Yorkshire): Association for Perioperative Practice; 2007.

98. Dumville JC, McFarlane E, Edwards P, et al. Preoperative skin antiseptics for preventing surgical wound infections after clean surgery. Cochrane Database Syst Rev 2015;(4):CD003949.

99. Yammine K, Harvey A. Efficacy of preparation solutions and cleansing techniques on contamination of the skin in foot and ankle surgery: a systematic review and meta-analysis. Bone Joint J 2013;95-B(4):498–503.

100. Scowcroft T. A critical review of the literature regarding the use of povidone iodine chlorhexidine gluconate for preoperative surgical skin preparation. J Perioper Pract 2012;22(3):95–9.

101. Ostrander RV, Botte MJ. Efficacy of surgical preparation solutions in foot and ankle surgery. J Bone Joint Surg Am 2005;87(5):980–5.

102. Keblish DJ. Preoperative skin preparation of the foot and ankle: bristles and alcohol are better. J Bone Joint Surg Am 2005;87(5):986–92.

103. Tachibana DK. Microbiology of the foot. Annu Rev Microbiol 1976;30:351–75.

104. Marshall J, Leeming JP, Holland KT. The cutaneous microbiology of normal human feet. J Appl Bacteriol 1987;62:139–46.

105. Zacharias J, Largen PS, Crosby LA. Results of preprocedure and postprocedure toe cultures in orthopaedic surgery. Foot Ankle Int 1998;19:166–8.

106. Bibbo C, Patel DV, Gehrmann RM, et al. Chlorhexidine provides superior skin decontamination in foot and ankle surgery. Clin Orthop Relat Res 2005;438:204–8.

107. Ostrander RV, Brage ME, Botte MJ. Bacterial skin contamination after surgical preparation in foot and ankle surgery. Clin Orthop Relat Res 2003;406:246–52.

108. Kumagai SG, Rosales RF, Hunter GC, et al. Effects of electrocautery on midline laparotomy wound infection. Am J Surg 1991;162:620–2.

109. Soballe PW, Nimbkar NV, Hayward I, et al. Electric cautery lowers the contamination threshold for infection of laparotomies. Am J Surg 1998;175:263–6.

110. Prakash LD, Balaji N, Kumar SS, et al. Comparison of electrocautery incision with scalpel incision in midline abdominal surgery – a double blind randomized controlled trial. Int J Surg 2015;19:78–82.

111. Babkin Y, Raveh D, Lifschitz M, et al. Incidence and risk factors for surgical infection after total knee replacement. Scand J Infect Dis 2007;39:890–5.

112. Anderson AE, Bergh I, Karlsson J, et al. Traffic flow in the operating room: an explorative and descriptive study on air quality during orthopedic trauma implant surgery. Am J Infect Control 2012;40(8):750–5.

113. Scaltriti S, Cencetti S, Rovesti S, et al. Risk factors for par¬ticulate and microbial contamination of air in operating theatres. J Hosp Infect 2007;66(4):320–6.

114. Mears SC, Blanding R, Belkoff SM. Door opening affects operating room pressure during joint arthroplasty. Orthopedics 2015;38(11):e991–4.

115. Hamilton WG, Balkam CB, Purcell RL, et al. Operating room traffic in total joint arthroplasty: Identifying patterns and training the team to keep the door shut. Am J Inf Control 2018;46:633–6.

116. Felippe WA, Werneck GL, Santoro-Lopes G. Surgical site infection among women discharged with a drain in situ after breast cancer surgery. World J Surg 2007;31:2293–9.

Periprocedural Concerns in the Patient with Renal Disease

Paris Payton, DPM[a],*, Ahmad Eter, MD[b]

KEYWORDS

- Nephrology • Chronic kidney disease • Perioperative concerns • Acute kidney injury

KEY POINTS

- Renal disease patients are at an overall higher risk of developing surgical complications.
- Renally compromised surgical patients need to be educated on potential surgical outcomes and complications, and they warrant a thorough preoperative evaluation including additional ancillary screening studies.
- Optimization of renal function, limitation of exposure to acute kidney injury, and utilization of adequate renal replacement therapy, when necessary, are essential for successful surgical outcomes in the renal patient.
- Nephrotoxic agents should be avoided in the perioperative setting to prevent further kidney injury and dysfunction.
- A multidisciplinary team approach to the perioperative management of the renal patient should be used.

INTRODUCTION

The dynamic function of the kidney and interaction with other organ systems places it in a critical role for physiology, compensatory mechanisms, and, ultimately, function of the human body. The renal system eliminates metabolic waste, regulates fluid and electrolyte homeostasis, and maintains acid-base homeostasis. In addition, the kidneys have endocrine functions that affect the cardiovascular and hematologic systems. Chronic kidney disease (CKD) is a pathologic process encompassing a broad spectrum of conditions that adversely affect renal function. This disease process involves the progressive loss of nephrons, inevitably resulting in end-stage renal disease (ESRD). The following is a list of acronyms and definitions used in this article:

Disclosure Statements: Drs P. Payton and A. Eter have no disclosures.
[a] St Vincent Charity Medical Center, 2351 East 22nd Street, Cleveland, OH 44115, USA;
[b] Nephrology, Princeton Community Hospital, 122 12th Street, Princeton, WV 24740, USA
* Corresponding author.
E-mail address: PPaytonDPM@gmail.com

- Chronic kidney disease (CKD)—progressively declining renal function secondary to a broad spectrum of conditions that adversely affect kidney function
- End-stage renal disease (ESRD)—in the absence of normal renal function, native kidney function must be replaced via dialysis or kidney transplantation
- Acute kidney injury (AKI)—previously known as acute renal failure (ARF), defined as an abrupt loss of kidney function usually over the course of approximately 7 days, generally caused by ischemic or inflammatory changes within the kidney, exposure to renally toxic substances, or an obstruction of the urinary tract impeding urine flow
- Glomerular filtration rate (GFR)
- Contrast-induced acute kidney injury (CI-AKI)—also referred to as contrast-induced nephropathy (CIN), defined as a decline in kidney function occurring in a narrow time window after administration of iodinated contrast material
- Contrast media (CM)
- Renal replacement therapy (RRT)—therapy that replaces the normal blood-filtering function of the kidneys
- Hemodialysis (HD)—medical procedure to remove fluid and waste products from the blood and to correct electrolyte imbalances
- Peritoneal dialysis (PT)—type of dialysis that uses the patient's own peritoneum as the membrane through which fluid and dissolved substances are filtered and exchanged with the blood

In the United States, the National Institute of Diabetes and Digestive and Kidney Diseases reports that 1 in 10 American adults has some level of CKD,[1] and that figure is projected to increase in the future with increasing prevalence of diabetes mellitus (DM) and cardiovascular disease. Thus, the frequency of this disease process coupled with the centrality of the kidney to normal homeostasis makes the management of impaired renal function a common and challenging problem in the perioperative setting. CKD can be associated with excess surgical morbidity, the most important of which include acute renal failure, hyperkalemia, volume overload, and infection.[2] The higher perioperative morbidity and mortality rates in patients who have renal disease, especially those with ESRD, reflect the importance of a properly functioning renal system.

CKD develops from several conditions including, but not limited to, DM, hypertension, glomerulonephropathy, renal vascular disease, obstructive uropathy, tubulointerstitial disease, as well as polycystic kidney disease. Renal function is evaluated by measuring glomerular filtration rate (GFR), which is expressed per 1.73 m^2 surface area because it is affected by age, sex, and body size. The average value of GFR for an adult man is 130 mL/min per 1.73 m^2 and is 120 mL/min per 1.73 m^2 for an adult woman.[3] CKD is defined by the National Kidney Foundation as either a GFR less than 60 mL/min/1.73 m^2 or kidney damage for more than or equal to 3 months. The term "kidney damage" denotes either anatomic abnormalities of the kidney or other markers of kidney damage, including abnormalities seen in the blood and urine or by imaging studies. The National Kidney Foundation-Kidney Disease Outcomes Quality Initiative (NKFK/DOQI) has proposed a standardized classification scheme for patients with CKD as outlined in **Table 1**. This classification scheme stratifies CKD into 5 stages based on estimation of GFR and documentation of renal injury. Patients with a GFR greater than 60 may also have CKD if there is evidence of abnormal pathology, imaging, or renal laboratory tests such as proteinuria for more than 3 months.[4] ESRD is defined as the need to replace native kidney function via dialysis or transplantation.

| Table 1 | | |
| Stages of chronic kidney disease | | |
Stage	Degree of Impairment	GFR (mL/min/1.73 m²)
1	Normal function, structural or genetic disposition	>90
2	Mildly reduced function with findings of Stage I	60–89
3	Moderately reduced function	30–59
4	Severely reduced function	15–29
5	End-stage renal disease or dialysis dependent	<15

Reprinted from American Journal of Kidney Diseases Vol 39, Issue 2, Part 4. Definition and Classi-fication of Stages of Chronic Kidney Disease, S46–S75, Copyright 2002, with permission from Elsevier.

ACUTE KIDNEY INJURY

Acute kidney injury (AKI), formerly known as acute renal failure, is a potential compli-cation of surgery in which the rapid loss of renal function over the course of days to weeks, resulting in the patient's inability to clear nitrogenous waste, including creati-nine and urea, from the body.[5] AKI during hospitalization increases morbidity, mortal-ity, length of stay, and cost of care.[6] Currently the RIFLE criteria are the most commonly used determinants for establishing the presence of AKI. RIFLE stands for risk, injury, failure, loss, and ESRD. The severity of kidney dysfunction increases across the letters of the acronym, from risk to ESRD. The categorization of the pa-tient's renal dysfunction is based on urine output and the change in serum creati-nine/percent decrease in GFR from baseline.

In the general population, the incidence of AKI after noncardiac surgery is low, and after orthopedic surgery the incidence is even lower, with reported rates often less than 1%.[7–9] Risk scores have been developed to predict the risk of AKI after cardiac surgery,[10] the risk of needing dialysis after cardiac surgery,[11] the risk of AKI in patients undergoing general surgery, and the risk of AKI following liver resection.[12] Unfortu-nately, no such risk scores exist in regard to orthopedic surgery.

Prevention is the most effective management of AKI, especially because there is no reliable way to reverse acute renal injury. Before surgery, the potential risk factors such as volume depletion, hypotension, sepsis, nephrotoxin exposure, and preexist-ing CKD should be identified. To prevent AKI, elective surgery should be postponed until those abnormalities are improved. However, treatment is merely supportive, decreasing the stress on the kidneys by avoiding hypotension and volume depletion, stopping nephrotoxic medications, correcting electrolyte imbalances and fluid over-load, and resorting to dialysis if needed. In the future, more sensitive biomarkers may replace serum creatinine in the diagnosis of AKI.[13] Biomarkers such as cystatin C, neutrophil gelatinase-associated lipocalin, kidney injury molecule-1, and others are currently being studied and may eventually enter clinical practice.[14]

PREOPERATIVE RENAL EVALUATION

The patient with renal disease requires a comprehensive preoperative evaluation, one that often encompasses several organ systems. As such, the coordination of care be-tween the foot and ankle specialist, nephrologist, anesthesiologist, and potentially other medical consultants is imperative. Management of preexisting renal disease may involve treating its underlying causes, managing the blood pressure, fluids and volume status, correcting electrolyte abnormalities, pharmacologic management, optimizing nutrition for surgical wound healing, and providing dialysis or transplant care. The ultimate goal is the assessment of the patient's risk for renal impairment with a given procedure and to institute measures directed at minimizing that risk. The typical preoperative diagnostic testing that should be performed in patients with CKD includes a renal panel, complete blood count, arterial blood gas measurements, bleeding time, chest radiograph as well as a physical examination with an emphasis on volume status.[15]

CKD is a risk factor for serious postoperative complications such as acute renal failure and cardiovascular complications, which are associated with increased morbidity and mortality.[16–18] During the preoperative evaluation, it is important to identify the risk factors for AKI and minimize them. Patients who suffer from an episode of AKI are at risk for a residual and progressive decline in kidney function, ESRD, and even death.[19–21] The greatest risk factor for such an outcome is preoperative CKD. Novis and colleagues,[18] in a systematic review of 28 heterogenous studies regarding preoperative risk factors for postoperative renal failure repeatedly, found that preoperative CKD was the only consistent risk factor for postoperative AKI.[7,15,22,23]

Unfortunately, in patients undergoing orthopedic surgery, patients with CKD often have multiple risk factors for AKI, including advanced age, obesity, as well as dysfunction in other major organ systems. Once identified, modifiable risk factors should be addressed if possible, because preventing postoperative AKI will improve both short- and long-term outcomes.[6] Cardiac and pulmonary function should be optimized. Nephrotoxins, hypotension, hypovolemia and hypervolemia should be avoided.

RENAL FUNCTION AND POSTOPERATIVE RISK

Surgical risk of patients with CKD, as in all patients, depends on the type of surgery and whether the procedure is routine or performed on an emergent basis. The extent of renal impairment and the necessity for dialysis in a patient also affects outcomes and subsequent morbidity of the proposed procedure. Myocardial infarction, heart failure, and stroke are the leading cause of death in patients with established renal failure.[24] Regardless of the cause, such patients often have coronary artery disease and, in fact, have a higher lifetime risk of death from cardiovascular disease than of ever-reaching ESRD.[25] Estimated morbidity rates for both cardiac and general surgery in patients with ESRD range from 14% to 64%.[15,26,27] Causes include decreased abilities to concentrate urine, regulate fluid volume and sodium concentrations, handle acid loads, and excrete potassium and medications. Hyperkalemia is the most frequent complication, followed by infection, hemodynamic instability, bleeding, and arrhythmias. Additional causes of morbidity include anemia, pericarditis, neuropathy, clotted vascular access ports, and infection.[15]

Although serum creatinine is the most widely used index of renal function in clinical practice, it is a relatively insensitive marker of renal function.[28] Serum creatinine is a function of both creatinine generation, primarily from muscle creatine metabolism, and renal and extrarenal creatinine excretion. Creatinine generation is proportional to muscle mass and is generally higher in men than in women and in individuals of African descent as compared with other racial groups. Furthermore, creatinine production tends to decline with increasing age and is also decreased in individuals with muscle wasting or malnutrition. Although creatinine excretion occurs primarily through glomerular filtration, a small percentage of creatinine is normally excreted by renal tubular secretion and in the stool. The percentage of creatinine excretion occurring via these nonglomerular routes increases with impaired renal function. As a consequence of these factors, serum creatinine concentration, particularly in elderly or chronically ill patients, may be normal or only minimally elevated despite significant reduction in GFR.

In order to improve the assessment of renal function from readily available clinical data, multiple prediction equations to estimate creatinine clearance and/or GFR have been developed. Calculating the patient's estimated GFR is the most appropriate and simplest way to determine the patient's renal risk. This value allows for appropriate medication dosing and establishes the degrees of risk for AKI, a risk that increases in a stepwise fashion with decreasing GFR. A 24-hour urine collection is the traditional standard of creatinine clearance determination (Equation 1).

Equation to estimate creatinine clearance and/or GFR

$$\text{Creatinine clearance (ml/minute)} = \frac{(140 - \text{age}) \times \text{weight(kg)}}{(72 \times \text{serum creatinine})} \times (0.85 \text{ if female})$$

Equation 1

This formula has not been validated in patients with stage I or II CKD and is applicable only when the serum creatinine is stable. In the setting of AKI, when the serum creatinine is rising, the estimated GFR is presumed to be less than 15 mL/min/1.73 m^2. Once the GFR has been established, recommendations are made to dose the patient's medications based on this value. The preoperative creatinine relative to historical values is also important. Patients with stable renal disease are at lower risk for worsening serum creatinine after surgery. Thus, in the patient with a progressively rising serum creatinine, elective procedures should be delayed until the cause of deteriorating renal function is identified and has been stabilized.

COMPLICATIONS OF RENAL IMPAIRMENT

When the excretory function of the kidney becomes impaired, an elevation in blood urea nitrogen levels, creatinine, and various protein metabolic products results. When there is impairment of the synthetic function of the kidney, decreased erythropoietin production results in anemia and decreased active vitamin D-3 causes hypocalcemia, secondary hyperparathyroidism, hyperphosphatemia, as well as renal osteodystrophy. Platelet dysfunction also results in excessive bleeding in the patient with CKD/ESRD. Synthetic dysfunction of the kidney also results in a reduction in acid, potassium, sodium chloride, and water excretion resulting in electrolyte disturbances including acidosis, hyperkalemia, hypertension, and edema. In addition, drugs normally excreted by the kidney can accumulate to toxic levels in patients with CKD; therefore, adjusting dosages or avoiding such drugs, including iodinated contrast in high-risk patients, is a key perioperative management principle in patients with CKD. The aforementioned complications must be identified and corrected perioperatively and early involvement of a nephrologist is strongly recommended to optimize outcomes and limit further kidney damage.

BLOOD PRESSURE, FLUID AND VOLUME MANAGEMENT

Volume-mediated hypertension is a common complication noted in patients with CKD and is oftentimes managed with diuretic therapy. Volume status should be assessed preoperatively and hypovolemia versus hypervolemia should be treated with volume or diuresis respectively to achieve a euvolemic state for surgery. Some patients with long-standing congestive heart failure (CHF) and concomitant kidney disease often demonstrate a "best" volume, which would mimic the euvolemic state. At this volume, heart and kidney function have achieved a physiologic balance allowing the highest level of function in this state.

In advanced chronic renal insufficiency, the ability to excrete even a modest sodium load is impaired and volume overload can rapidly develop following administration of only small quantities of enteral or intravenous (IV) fluids. Lactated Ringer solution is generally avoided in renal patients due to its potassium content resulting in the propensity for hyperkalemia.[28] Because of their inability to excrete excess fluid content, administration of large volumes of IV fluids should be avoided in patients with CKD/ESRD due to the risk of volume overload. If volume overload develops, IV fluids should be discontinued and diuretic therapy using furosemide or bumetanide should be initiated. In patients with ESRD, volume overload may precipitate the need for urgent dialysis.

Paradoxically, patients with mild to moderate CKD are also at increased risk for the development of extracellular fluid volume depletion. A sudden decrease in sodium intake or increased extrarenal losses due to diarrhea, nasogastric suction, vomiting, enterocutaneous fistulas, burns, or fever may therefore be associated with relative renal "salt-wasting" and clinically significant volume depletion. This volume depletion may be exacerbated further by the inadvisable use of diuretics.

Because patients with CKD are at risk for both volume depletion and volume overload, the IV fluid rate should account for insensible losses, residual urine output, and anticipated blood loss with additional IV fluid boluses as needed. Central hemodynamic monitoring is frequently necessary to guide fluid management, especially in patients with concomitant cardiac or hepatic dysfunction.[28]

ELECTROLYTE DISTURBANCES

Hyponatremia and hyperkalemia are sometimes encountered during preoperative laboratory testing. The cause should be determined and appropriate treatment administered, based on the results of the workup. Although there are no values of serum sodium or potassium that are considered totally safe before surgery, some observations can be made. The safety of any given serum sodium is likely related to the cause of the hyponatremia, its chronicity, and the patient's symptoms (if any). Clinical experience also suggests that patients with CKD, especially ESRD, tolerate hyperkalemia better than the general population. Indeed, in one study, electrocardiographic changes occurred only at a serum potassium level greater than 6.5 mmol/L.[29]

Hyperkalemia may be precipitated by tissue breakdown, transfusions, acidosis, and angiotensin-converting enzyme (ACE) inhibitors, beta-blockers, heparin, rhabdomyolysis, and the use of potassium-containing lactated Ringer solution as a replacement fluid. In patients with an elevated serum potassium but not obvious cause, ruling out "pseudohyperkalemia" by checking concurrent plasma potassium is reasonable. Once confirmed, all patients presenting with hyperkalemia should promptly be switched to a low potassium diet. The patient's current medications should be reviewed for any agents that may precipitate an increase in serum potassium levels. Such medications should be held or supplemented by an alternative agent if possible.

If echocardiogram (ECG) changes are noted, an infusion of calcium salts, calcium gluconate, or calcium chloride should immediately be implemented to decrease the potassium level.[30] Recent literature suggests that calcium should be administered when the serum potassium concentration is greater than 6.0 to 6.5 mmol/L, even in the absence of ECG abnormalities.[30] Agents that transiently shift potassium intracellularly, such as albuterol, bicarbonate, and dextrose with insulin, should also be implemented, and use of a loop diuretic will also result in potassium excretion, thus lowering serum potassium levels. Bicarbonate infusion is the most reliable treatment for acute hyperkalemia after calcium salt infusion.[30] Combination therapy with insulin and salbutamol has a synergistic effect and is accepted as a safe treatment in patients with ESRD. Emergency dialysis may be required in the case of severe and treatment-resistant hyperkalemia. In any case, frequent electrolyte checks are necessary to monitor the abnormalities during the perioperative period.

ANEMIA

The kidneys are responsible for the production of erythropoietin; therefore, as renal function declines patients are likely to develop anemia.[31] Although there is no published standard for safe preoperative hematocrit levels in patients with impaired renal function, one study[26] demonstrated increased intraoperative complications in patients with ESRD and preoperative hematocrit levels ranging from 20% to 26%. Associated with an increased mortality in CKD,[32] the presence of anemia also correlates with higher mortality in patients undergoing cardiac[33,34] and noncardiac surgery.[35] In one orthopedic study, however, the patients' comorbidities rather than their preoperative anemia correlated best with postoperative complications and mortality.[36]

Correcting severe or hemodynamically significant anemia may help to avoid complications from perioperative blood loss. Before the widespread use of erythropoietin-stimulating agents (ESAs), patients with CKD required transfusions to treat their anemia, which oftentimes resulted in hyperkalemia. Nonautologous blood transfusions should also be limited or avoided because they lead to antibody formation that will ultimately decrease the likelihood of successful renal transplantation in the future. Even today under some circumstances blood transfusion may be necessary; however, if the surgery is elective, ESAs may be administered to maintain a hematocrit of at least 30 before surgery. Treatment should be initiated several weeks before surgery, so that the hormone has adequate time to increase the hematocrit to the desired level. Iron stores should also be checked in all patients receiving erythropoietin. For maximum effectiveness of erythropoietin, iron deficiency should be remedied with oral supplements. These recommendations are fairly similar to those for the treatment of preoperative anemia before elective surgeries such as joint replacements.[37]

UREMIC BLEEDING

Uremia can cause platelet dysfunction, which can result in increased perioperative bleeding. To minimize uremic complications, patients with ESRD should undergo dialysis on the day before surgery. Bleeding time is a standard test that should be obtained perioperatively in the renal disease patient because it is the most sensitive indicator of the degree of platelet dysfunction. Although bleeding times greater than 10 to 15 minutes have been associated with a high risk of hemorrhage,[38] the exact correction of elevated bleeding times and surgical risk has not been clearly established.

Desmopressin acetate can enhance hemostasis in general[39] and specifically improve the platelet dysfunction in uremia.[40] Despite an extensive published record, the use of desmopressin for uremic patients undergoing surgery remains controversial. One review article[39] and a Cochrane review[41] did not support the use of desmopressin to reduce blood loss and decrease transfusion requirements. However, another meta-analysis[42] did find a small but statistically significant reduction in blood loss and blood transfusion requirement although the percentage of patients who received transfusions was not changed. Desmopressin acetate is not approved by Food and Drug Administration for hemostasis; however, when given for this indication, the dose is usually 0.3 mcg/kg IV, with a maximum of 20mcg. Side effects include flushing, hyponatremia, myocardial infarction or other thrombotic events, and hypotension; however, in the meta-analysis by Crescenzi and colleagues,[42] only clinically insignificant hypotension occurred more often in patients receiving desmopressin as compared with the placebo group. In most studies, patients were included regardless of severity of kidney disease, so it is possible that desmopressin may be more beneficial in the uremic patient. Standard options for correcting an elevated bleeding time include intensive dialysis, desmopressin (DDAVP, 0.3 mcg/kg, IV 1 hour before surgery[43]), cryoprecipitate (10u over 30 minutes IV; effects should be apparent in 1 hour[44]), conjugated estrogens (0.6 mg/kg per day IV or orally for 5 days; some effect should be apparent in 6 hours, but peak effect occurs in 5–7 days), and packed red blood cell transfusion.[45]

Antiplatelet agents, including aspirin and dipyridamole, should not be administered within 72 hours of surgery in patients with CKD/ESRD. In addition, some agents that typically only affect platelets minimally in patients without uremia can have exaggerated effects in patients with ESRD and may theoretically increase the risk of intraoperative bleeding. These drugs include diphenhydramine, nonsteroidal antiinflammatory drugs (NSAIDs), chlordiazepoxide, and cimetidine.[45]

PHARMACOLOGIC MANAGEMENT

Choosing which medications to hold before surgery in order to decrease the chance of AKI remains controversial; however, several classes of drugs are believed to be especially problematic in the patient with kidney disease. For example, NSAIDs, even cyclooxygenase-2 inhibitors, negatively affect the kidney function by impairing renal autoregulation through a mechanism that inhibits prostaglandin-mediated dilation of the afferent arteriole in the glomerulus.[46] Consequently, NSAIDs should be avoided in the perioperative setting due to their nephrotoxic potential and alternative agents of analgesia should be implemented instead. Further, ACE inhibitors and angiotensin II receptor blockers (ARBs) diminish the ability of the afferent arteriole to constrict[46] and are reported to cause hypotension during the induction phase of anesthesia.[13,47] A meta-analysis supported this finding but found insufficient data to draw conclusions about other outcomes, such as AKI.[48] However, in one study,[49] ACE inhibitor or ARB therapy combined with diuretics increased the risk of hypotension and in another study increased the risk of AKI, although reported solely in bariatric surgery.[50] Reasonable recommendations from a review on perioperative medication management suggest holding ACE inhibitors and ARBs for patients who take these medications for hypertension and have acceptably controlled blood pressure.[51] In short, patients with CKD should generally hold NSAIDs, ACE inhibitors, ARBs, and diuretics in the morning of orthopedic surgery. Patients who take such medications for treatment of CHF may need to continue their medication perioperatively, and in such circumstances, the patient's cardiologist should be consulted for an individualized approach to pharmacologic therapy. All medications held preoperatively should be considered for reinitiation postoperatively once hemodynamic stability and euvolemia are achieved.

USE OF CONTRAST WHEN IMAGING PATIENTS WITH RENAL DISEASE

Medical imaging has become an important diagnostic and therapeutic tool in preparation for surgery. Contrast media (CM) are increasingly used for better imaging in a broad spectrum of areas such as diagnostic angiography, computed tomography (CT) and MRI, peripheral interventional endovascular procedures, diagnostic cardiac catheterization, and of interventional percutaneous transluminal coronary angioplasty (PTCA). Imaging the renal patient can present significant challenges particularly when the preferred imaging modality requires the use of contrast. Contrast-induced acute kidney injury (CI-AKI) is one of the most common causes of AKI in clinical practice, and recent studies have demonstrated that both short-term and long-term mortality rates are significantly higher in patients with CI-AKI as compared with those without CI-AKI.[52] Further, a history of CI-AKI may be associated with preexisting CKD and long-term progression to ESRD.[53,54] Because of the risk and severity of this condition, a serum creatinine and estimation of GFR should be determined in all patients undergoing radiologic studies with contrast.

The most widely used definition of CI-AKI is the increase in serum creatinine greater than 0.5 mg/dL or 25% increase of serum creatinine from the baseline value at 48 hours after CM administration. For renal insufficiency to be attributable to contrast administration, it should be acute, usually occurring within 2 to 3 days. However, it has been suggested that renal insufficiency developing up to 7 days post–contrast administration can be considered contrast-induced nephropathy (CIN). Following contrast exposure, serum creatinine levels peak between 2 and 5 days and usually return to normal in 14 days. Because the use of serum creatinine as a marker of renal function has its limitations, indicators such as the estimated GFR and cystatin C levels have been considered as alternative and reliable reflectors of existing renal function.[55,56] In a study, by Briguori and colleagues,[57] performed on patients with CKD undergoing PTCA, increased cystatin C levels greater than or equal to 10% at 24 hours after the procedure was found to reliably predict patients at high risk of CI-AKI.

CI-AKI is normally a transient process, with renal function reverting to normal within 7 to 14 days of contrast administration. Less than one-third of patients develop some degree of residual renal impairment, although this value is increased in diabetics and those with preexisting renal disease. The incidence of CI-AKI in patients undergoing elective, nonemergent contrast-enhanced CT has been found to be less than 1%.[58] In patients with CKD, the incidence of CI-AKI after IV CM administration was found to be 4%.[59] However, the incidence of CI-AKI following contrast-enhanced CT performed in an emergent setting was found to be greater than 10%, which suggests the increased vulnerability of critically ill patients to CI-AKI. In a study performed on critically ill patients without preexisting renal disease, serum creatinine levels were elevated to greater than 25% from baseline in 18% of patients following CM-enhanced CT.[60]

The size and number of organic molecules binding the iodine are the primary determinant of the ionicity, osmolarity, and viscosity of the media. High-osmolarity contrast media (HOCM) have an iodine to molecule ratio of 1.5:1; low-osmolarity, nonionic contrast media (LOCM) have an iodine to molecule ratio of 3:1; and iso-osmolar contrast media (IOCM) have an iodine to molecule ratio of 6:1.[61] Hyperosmolar CM (HOCM) has been demonstrated more frequently to cause CI-AKI as compared with low-osmolar CM (LOCM).[62] Kidney Disease Improving Global Outcomes (KDIGO) guidelines recommend use of LOCM or IOCM instead of HOCM,[63] which is no longer used in clinical practice. Recent meta-analyses[64,65] found that iodixanol (IOCM) was found to be associated with a reduced risk of CI-AKI as compared with LOCM; however, in these studies no significant difference was found between IOCM and LOCM in terms of renal safety. IOCM has lower osmolality compared with LOCM but has greater viscosity due to its dimeric structure as compared with the monomeric structure of LOCM. Viscosity rather than osmolality determines resistance to blood flow, thus IOCM may impair renal medullary blood flow to a greater extent than LOCM, exacerbating medullary hypoxia.[66,67] Thus, because of a lack of conclusive evidence,

KDIGO guidelines do not make a recommendation about the preference of IOCM versus LOCM.[63] Lower doses of CM (definitions of low dose are variable: <30– 125 mL) were found to be less nephrotoxic.[68,69] Recently, newer CT modalities have been developed using low tube voltage and low CM volume to reduce radiation exposure as well as the risk of CI-AKI without sacrificing image quality.[70–72] However, even very low doses of CM may lead to CI-AKI in patients with multiple risk factors.

Ultrasound CT scan without IV contrast, and MRI without gadolinium are all safe for renal patients. The gadolinium-based contrast agents (GBCA) used in MRI were previously believed to be safe in terms of nephrotoxicity. However, in patients with preexisting CKD and diabetic nephropathy, these agents have also been reported to cause AKI, especially at the high doses used in angiography.[73–75] In an in vitro study, cytotoxicity of GBCA was compared with that of iodinated CM in renal tubular cells at angiographic concentrations and GBCA was not less cytotoxic compared with iomeprol.[76] These results suggest that GBCA also induces cytotoxicity in renal tubular cells. Another important adverse effect of GBCA is nephrogenic systemic fibrosis (NSF), which occurs especially in patients with CKD and can be a potentially fatal complication. GBCA should be avoided in patients with ESRD due to the increased risk of NSF. If it is inevitable to use GBCA in patients with ESRD, immediate hemodialysis (HD) after the imaging procedure should be considered because GBCA has been shown to be effectively removed by HD.[77] In HD patients without urine output, if contrast-enhanced imaging is required, CT is preferred over MRI to avoid the risk of NSF.

Patients who are scheduled to have a contrast-enhanced diagnostic or interventional procedure should be evaluated for risk factors of CI-AKI, the most important being preexisting CKD and DM with diabetic nephropathy. In a study performed on patients undergoing contrast-enhanced CT, incidence of CI-AKI was found to be higher in patients with diabetic CKD as compared with those with nondiabetic CKD.[78] Several risk scoring systems have been developed to predict CI-AKI. Mehran and colleagues[79] proposed a CI-AKI risk stratification score based on 8 readily available variables, including (1) patient-related features such as age greater than 75 years, DM, chronic CHF, acute pulmonary edema, hypotension, anemia, and CKD; and (2) procedure-related features such as the use of intraaortic balloon pump or increasing volumes of CM. Integer scores were given to these risk factors as outlined in **Table 2**.

These scores are summed for a total risk score. For example, if the total risk score is less than or equal to 5, risk of CI-AKI is 7.5% and risk of dialysis is 0.04%. However, with a total risk score of greater than or equal to 16, risk of CI-AKI is 57% and risk of dialysis is 13%.[79] Mehran's study determined that increasing total risk score exponentially predicts increased risk of CI-AKI. The ACEF score composed of age, creatinine, and ejection fraction is another simple risk scoring system for CI-AKI in patients undergoing percutaneous transluminal coronary angioplasty and has been found to be an independent and useful predictor of CI-AKI defined as an increase in serum creatinine greater than or equal to 0.5 mg/dL.[80,81]

There is no specific treatment for CI-AKI, thus prevention is the cornerstone of CIN management, and hydration therapy is the cornerstone of CIN prevention. Similar to the management of other types of AKI, stabilization of hemodynamic parameters and maintenance of normal fluid and electrolyte balance is crucial. Renal perfusion is decreased for up to 20 hours following contrast administration. Intravascular volume expansion maintains renal blood flow, preserves nitric oxide production, prevents medullary hypoxemia, and enhances contrast elimination. The best preventative measure of CI-AKI is to avoid unnecessary contrast

Table 2
Risk factors of contrast-induced acute kidney injury

Risk Factor	Score
Hypotension	5
IABP	5
CHF	5
Age >75 y	4
Anemia	3
DM	3
Serum creatinine >1.5 mg/dL	4
Each 100 mL of CM	1
eGFR = 40–60 mL/min per 1.73 m^2	2
eGFR = 20–40 mL/min per 1.73 m^2	4
eGFR <20 mL/min per 1.73 m^2	6

Abbreviations: eGFR, estimated glomerular filtration rate; IABP, intraaortic balloon pump.
From Mehran R, Aymong ED, Nikolsky E, et al. A simple risk score for prediction of contrast-induced nephropathy after percutaneous coronary intervention: development and initial validation. J Am Coll Cardiol 2004;44:1393–9; with permission.

administration, which requires a good communication between the clinician and the radiologist/interventionalist. Alternative imaging modalities should always be considered; however, if contrast use is inevitable, minimizing the amount of contrast, using iso-osmolar nonionic contrast agents, and administration of the antioxidant acetylcysteine should be implemented to reduce the risk of CI-AKI. Any concomitant use of nephrotoxic drugs such as NSAIDs should be discontinued before the procedure. Preemptive HD or hemofiltration has not shown to be of any benefit and is not recommended.[82]

Several therapies for treatment and/or prevention of CI-AKI have been investigated; however, intravascular hydration seems to be the best preventative measure.[80,83–86] Prevention focuses on avoiding volume depletion, which has led to trials and practices using oral hydration, volume expansion with IV fluids and bicarbonate, and both holding and using diuretics. Treatment is mainly supportive and aimed at volume and electrolyte balance. Some patients may require renal replacement therapy, but this need is usually transient. Sodium bicarbonate and N-acetylcysteine (NAC) have been investigated for their protective effects against AKI and both have had supportive evidence for success. The efficacy of these supplemental treatments is still debated throughout the literature. However, in 2012, KDIGO suggested NAC for patients with high risk of CI-AKI[63] because it is generally well tolerated and inexpensive with a relatively good profile of adverse effects. A systematic review and meta-analysis of prevention strategies for CIN found that, compared with IV saline only, the following had clinically important and statistically significant benefits when used in combination with IV saline[87]: (1) low-dose NAC with a risk ratio (RR) of 0.75, (2) NAC in patients receiving LOCM with an RR of 0.69, (3) statins plus NAC with an RR of 0.52.

New alternative noncontrast-enhanced imaging modalities have been developed in recent years, most of these modalities being MRI-based techniques. Knowledge of these new techniques may be beneficial for the renal health of the patients needing contrast-enhancing imaging and interventions. These new modalities and their indications are detailed in **Table 3**.

Table 3
Alternative noncontrast-enhanced imaging techniques

Name of Technique	Clinical Indications	Misc.
TOF MR angiography	Cerebral aneurysm Stroke Atherosclerotic carotid disease Arteriovenous malformation Peripheral arterial disease	No contrast agent required
ECG-gated fast spin echo MR angiography	Peripheral arterial disease Thoracoabdominal aortic aneurysm	No contrast agent required Higher image quality compared with TOF MR angiography in peripheral arterial imaging
SSFP MRI	Coronary artery disease Myocardial viability and function Pericardial diseases Renal artery stenosis Congenital heart disease	No contrast agent required
Arterial spin labeling with/without SSFP	Native and transplanted renal artery stenosis Renal perfusion Cerebral blood flow Characterization of masses	No contrast agent required Evaluation of organ perfusion When combined with SSFP, it can be used as angiographic imaging
Phase-contrast MRI	Imaging of major thoracoabdominal vessels Congenital heart disease Renal artery stenosis	No contrast agent required Quantification of blood flow and velocity
Carbon-dioxide angiography	Peripheral artery disease (mostly infradiaphragmatic)	No contrast agent required Nonallergenic, nonnephrogenic, inexpensive, neurotoxic Risk of air trapping and distal ischemia

Abbreviations: SSFP, steady-state free precession; TOF, time of flight.
From Ozkok S, Ozkok A. Contrast-induced acute kidney injury: a review of practical points. World J Nephrol 2017;6(3):86–99; with permission.

ANALGESIA

NSAIDs should be avoided in patients with CKD, especially those with other risk factors for AKI. In circumstances where NSAIDs must be given, the dosage should be limited. Meperidine and propoxyphene should also be avoided due to the toxic effects of their metabolites, which accumulate in patients with CKD.[88] The pharmacologically active metabolites of morphine also have a prolonged half-life, and the dose of morphine required to achieve pain relief in patients with CKD is usually lower than in patients with normal renal function. One source[89] has recommended fentanyl and methadone as the opiates of choice in CKD and dialysis patients, although these narcotics are the least dialyzable if the patient develops an adverse side effect.[90]

WOUND CARE

Impaired renal function has long been recognized to have implications on wound healing. The adverse effects of uremia on fibroblast proliferation, hydroxyproline level, and collagen production in wounds were identified as early as the 1960s and 1970s.[91–93] Although there have been limited human studies on the effects of wound healing in uremic patients, animal models have clearly demonstrated that the addition of urea or uremic serum inhibits fibroblast growth and delays wound healing.[93] Research data on mice suggest that the effect of CKD on wound healing is mediated by the disruption of keratinization kinetics, the delayed rate of granulation, and a large epithelial gap. The underlying chronic inflammatory state and low rate of vascularization and cell proliferation were also identified as mechanisms that lead to poor wound healing.[94] Rats with renal failure have been shown to form less granulation tissue than those with normal kidney function.[95] Supporting the animal data, human research has confirmed that patients with CKD have a higher rate of wound disruption than individuals with normal GFR.[96] Pollard and colleagues[97] showed a significant correlation between ESRD and the failure of transmetatarsal amputations to heal. Further, according to a recently published surgical bypass study,[98] the wound healing rate was approximately 60% to 80% at 1 year in patients with ESRD as compared with approximately 90% in non-ESRD patients. Another study by Kawarada and colleagues,[99] evaluating the impact of ESRD in patients with critical limb ischemia undergoing infrapopliteal intervention, demonstrated that patients with ESRD had lower patency of the pedal arch and were at approximately twice the risk of wound healing failure, reintervention, and death or major amputation than non-ESRD patients.

In the early stages of CKD (stages 1–3), impairment of renal function can manifest as proteinuria and variable edema, whereas in stage 4 to 5 CKD, substantial edema, electrolyte abnormalities, acid-base disorders, and secondary hyperparathyroidism often develop. All these factors and the uremic toxins present in patients with CKD at various stages of the disease are important considerations with regard to the aspects of surgical site healing. Variable levels of zinc have also been reported in patients with uremia.[100] Zinc is an imperative element for wound healing because it serves as a cofactor in a zinc-dependent pathway that augments autodebridement and keratinocyte migration. Zinc also confers protection against reactive oxygen species and bacterial toxins that impede wound healing. As discussed earlier, chronic renal patients often suffer from iron deficiency and anemia of chronic disease. Anemia is associated with poor tissue oxygenation and impaired wound healing. The iron repletion commonly needed in patients with ESRD to optimize erythropoiesis may also inadvertently impair wound healing in these individuals. Iron overload not only compromises the immune system but also causes the inhibited synthesis and release of vascular endothelial growth factor (VEGF), which helps maintain angiogenesis. Recent evidence suggests that iron depletion with deferoxamine improves tissue oxygenation and facilitates wound healing by abrogating iron-mediated impairment of VEGF upregulation.[101] Patients with CKD are also frequently volume-overloaded, leading to significant lower extremity edema, which acts as another barrier to healing.

Several uremic toxins have also been investigated for their implications on surgical site and wound healing in the patient with CKD. Some of these toxins are water soluble and easily removed via dialysis, whereas others are strongly protein bound or have a high molecular weight and therefore cannot be removed using dialysis.[102] One specifically interesting uremic toxin is beta-2 microglobulin, which is a large and poorly dialyzable molecule. Accumulation of beta-2 microglobulin leads to the development of systemic amyloidosis in dialysis patients, which in turn has a wide spectrum of manifestations, including bone fractures, carpal tunnel syndrome, and polyneuropathy. In terms of mechanism of action, some toxins exhibit adverse effects on wound healing via platelet dysfunction and impaired hemostasis, whereas others, such as interleukin 6, contribute to the chronic inflammatory state. Accumulation of asymmetric dimethylarginine interferes with L-arginine action and leads to the generation of nitric oxide and impaired endothelial function.[103] Further, excess 3-deoxyglucosone (a precursor for advanced glycosylation products) contributes to impaired collagen function, among other abnormalities.

Peripheral arterial disease (PAD) is another common comorbidity in patients with kidney disease, especially those on hemodialysis. Not only is vascular insufficiency 3 times more prevalent in individuals with CKD than in those without, but the severity of PAD worsens with increased severity of CKD.[104] Patients with CKD are highly predisposed to accelerated atherosclerotic plaque formation because of the presence of not only the traditional risk factors for peripheral vascular disease but also other CKD-specific risk factors such as chronic inflammation, malnutrition, fluid retention, alterations in the renin-angiotensin system, hyperhomocysteinemia, abnormal mineral metabolism, dyslipidemia, lipoprotein imbalances, and oxidative stress.[105] The overall prevalence of PAD among adult hemodialysis and peritoneal dialysis patients has been reported to be 25% and 19%, respectively.[106] It has also been shown that 24% of adults older than 40 years with a creatinine clearance of less than 60 mL/min had an ankle brachial index of less than 0.9.[107] However, vascular calcification that is seen in more than one-third of the ESRD population may influence the accuracy of these results.

Vascular calcification occurs in CKD because as renal function decreases, phosphate clearance is reduced and hyperphosphatemia results. Calcium and phosphorus are deposited within the vascular bed, leading to vascular calcification. ESRD is also associated with elevated levels of parathyroid hormone, which has been linked to vascular calcification.[108] In addition to vascular calcification, chronic inflammation demonstrated by chronically elevated C-reactive protein (CRP) significantly increases the risk of atherosclerosis. Ridker and colleagues[109] showed that CRP levels were found to be significantly higher in patients who developed symptomatic PAD as compared with controls.

CRP levels have been shown to be elevated in approximately one-third of all hemodialysis patients.[110] Hemodialysis itself has been shown to cause a drop in microvascular blood flow, worsen underlying PAD, impair wound healing, and reduce transcutaneous oxygen tension during and for several hours after dialysis.[111] It is thought that huge fluid shifts and the resultant hemodynamic changes during dialysis are responsible for the dialysis-mediated tissue hypoperfusion. Although hyperbaric oxygen therapy has improved wound healing in diabetics, less of a response has been seen in patients with renal failure. Only 58% of patients with renal failure improved after hyperbaric oxygen treatment, compared with 76% of patients without renal failure.[112]

Although it is known that patients with renal failure have an impaired immune system and are predisposed to infections, little is known about the mechanism of this immune imbalance. The effect of uremic toxins inciting chronic inflammation in severe kidney disease has been reported to alter the inflammatory response to surgical site healing as well as compromise many aspects of the immune system, making these patients more susceptible to infection. Uremia causes hyporeactive monocytes, depressed bactericidal action of neutrophils, compromised complement activation, diminished T and B lymphocyte function, a reduction in natural killer cell activity, and impaired function of polymorphonuclear cells, the main cells that fight bacterial infections.[113] Elevated levels of iron and calcium, anemia from chronic renal disease, and hemodialysis have all been shown to further exacerbate disorders in polymorphonuclear cell function.[114] In 2008, Foley reported that the septicemia-related mortality was 100 to 300 times higher in dialysis patients than in a matched cohort from the general population.[115] Unfortunately, clinical trials providing information on the outcomes of postsurgical infection in patients with renal failure are scarce. Animal research on mice with surgically induced CKD showed that these mice had a similar rate of postsurgical wound infection as a control group with preserved renal function, although wound healing was delayed in the former group.[116] In addition, the presence of a hemodialysis catheter or a synthetic vascular graft is a risk factor for systemic infection. Collectively, the findings seem to indicate that clinicians should consider the risk of development of systemic infection as well as local wound infection to be higher in patients with renal impairment.

Surgical site healing is also largely affected by nutrition status, which is oftentimes compromised in severe renal disease patients. Malnutrition has been reported to be present in 40% to 70% of patients with ESRD.[117] Many health care providers are unaware that renal replacement therapy (RRT) in the form of hemodialysis or peritoneal dialysis predisposes patients to significant protein loss. It has been reported that hemodialysis patients lose 6 to 8 g of amino acids per procedure, whereas peritoneal dialysis patients lose 8 to 20 g of protein per day from the peritoneal cavity. This loss of protein and the ensuing protein-deficient state have a significant negative impact on wound healing.[118] The criteria used for the diagnosis of protein-energy wasting are serum albumin less than 3.8 g/L, serum prealbumin less than 30 mg/dL, and serum cholesterol less than 100 mg/dL.[119] Low serum albumin levels have also been associated with poor wound healing.[120] In addition, some patients on dialysis may have decreased albumin synthesis due to underlying inflammatory process regardless of adequate nutrition. Prealbumin, unlike albumin, has a short half-life and changes rapidly in response to alterations in nutritional status. Decreased prealbumin levels are correlated independently with increased mortality and hospitalization due to infection.[120]

Nutritional supplementation of protein in dialysis patients is very important. Several protein-containing supplemental products have been designed specifically for patients with kidney disease, and a distinct feature of these products is their low potassium ($\leq$200 mg) and phosphorus ($\leq$150 mg) content, which is essential in patients who have impaired renal excretion of these electrolytes. Minerals such as zinc, selenium, and iron can also be removed with dialysis and should be supplemented in specific renal doses. The use of multivitamin complexes designed specifically for renal failure patients along with a multidisciplinary approach should be used to promote surgical site healing and achieve favorable outcomes during the postoperative course.

RENAL REPLACEMENT THERAPY: DIALYSIS AND TRANSPLANTATION

When preparing a patient with ESRD for surgery, special consideration must be given to the patient's dialysis or transplant needs. A nephrologist must be involved in coordinating this care.

Hemodialysis Patients

For patients already on dialysis, the following need to be determined[90]: (1) dialysis adequacy, (2) preoperative dialysis needs, (3) postoperative dialysis timing, and (4) dosage requirements for all medications. Patients on hemodialysis, including peritoneal dialysis, usually require preoperative dialysis within 24 hours before surgery to reduce the risks of volume overload, hyperkalemia, and excessive bleeding. Ideally, an HD patient should receive dialysis the night before surgery, even if this alters the patient's regular three-times-per-week schedule. This renders the patient's blood as "clean" as possible for surgery. Repeat laboratories should not be drawn within the first few hours following hemodialysis, because the electrolytes may be falsely low, having not yet reequilibrated. For this reason, supplemental potassium should never be given based on laboratories drawn in the immediate postdialysis period. The well-dialyzed patient should also experience fewer uremic complications such as poor platelet function and delayed wound healing. In addition, preoperative dialysis usually delays the need for dialysis after surgery. This is particularly beneficial in those patients who are not hemodynamically stable in the early postoperative period.[28]

Sufficient fluid is generally removed to make the patient euvolemic and achieve the patient's dry weight (the patient's target weight at the end of dialysis). A small amount of heparin is used during hemodialysis, with a residual anticoagulant effect lasting as long as 1.5 to 2 hours. The effect of this heparin on intraoperative bleeding is not clear. Traditionally, no heparin is used during the final preoperative HD session and unless heparin-free dialysis is used, it is prudent to wait at least 12 hours after the last hemodialysis with heparin before performing an invasive surgical procedure.[121] The use of heparin with dialysis is also avoided for at least 1 to 2 days following major orthopedic surgery. However, many orthopedic procedures require anticoagulation after surgery and thus would require patients to receive heparin-free dialysis anyway.

Vascular access including arteriovenous fistula (AVF), arteriovenous graft (AVG), or a tunneled HD catheter is required to perform HD. Because maintaining a functioning vascular access is critically important, special attention must be given to the access. All blood pressures, blood draws, and IVs should be performed on the contralateral extremity to the functioning AVF or AVG[90] because using the arm with the HD access increases risk of thrombosis and fistula/graft malfunction. In fact, IV placement should be limited to only what is absolutely necessary in order to preserve the patient's other veins for further HD access placement.

Any required central venous catheter should be placed also contralateral to the HD access; otherwise the HD access may not function as well.[28] The internal jugular location for catheters is preferred over the subclavian location due to the risk of subclavian stenosis and decreased function of the current (or future) access in the ipsilateral arm. Providers obtaining central venous access in an HD patient should be aware that patients with long-standing history of HD may have one or more occluded central veins from current or previous central venous catheters, cardiac pacemakers, or other injuries and procedures.

An existing tunneled dialysis catheter should not be used during surgery unless no other IV access can be obtained. The catheter traditionally had an anticoagulant (usually heparin) dwelling in the tubing in order to decrease the chance of thrombosis. In patients with advanced CKD who are approaching ESRD and the need for dialysis, one should avoid using the nondominant arm for blood pressure readings, blood draws, and IVs, if possible, because HD access will likely be created in this arm in the future.

Peritoneal Dialysis Patients

Peritoneal dialysis (PD) is a form of renal replacement therapy in which the clearance of toxins and ultrafiltration of water take place via the peritoneal membrane by exchanging substances from blood to PD fluid and vice versa. The patient either manually exchanges fluid in the peritoneal cavity an average of 4 times daily or uses a cycler to exchange the fluid at night while sleeping. When a PD patient undergoes a surgical procedure, alterations in the dialysis schedule are also needed. Some nephrologists recommend performing PD exchanges more frequently before surgery, but the beneficial effect of this strategy on surgical outcomes is not clear. PD patients should be advised to drain the fluid from their abdomen on the morning of surgery. A dry abdomen during surgery should be tolerated by a regularly dialyzed patient and will have only a small effect on electrolyte and fluid balance. In contrast, leaving PD fluid in the abdomen increases intraabdominal pressure[28] and leads to the absorption of fluid during surgery, thus risking fluid overload.

Assuming that the peritoneum was not compromised during surgery, PD can usually be resumed the morning after surgery (barring any emergent electrolyte or fluid issues requiring earlier initiation), when the patient is more alert and able to assist with the fluid exchanges. PD patients do not have the same dietary restrictions as patients receiving hemodialysis. For example, although phosphorus and total fluid intake should be limited, potassium restriction is usually not necessary due to the nearly continuous removal of potassium provided by this form of dialysis. However, PD patients should still have their potassium level followed; if lower, they can be encouraged to increase oral potassium intake or receive small doses of potassium repletion.

Renal Transplant Patients

Because of complicated interactions and immunosuppressive dosing, monitoring, and adjustment, a nephrologist with specialized knowledge of renal transplantation should be involved in the preoperative evaluation of patients with CKD who have received kidney transplantation. Renal transplant patients should continue their regular immunosuppressive medications up to, and including, the morning of surgery. As soon as feasible after surgery, the patient should be allowed to continue taking their regular transplant medications orally. If oral administration is not possible, administration via nasogastric tube should be considered. If the transplant medication cannot be given enterally, IV formulation may be given as long as it is dosed appropriately. A nephrologist or pharmacist experienced in transplant medications should assist with the conversion of outpatient medications to an IV equivalent.

Calcineurin inhibitors such as cyclosporine or tacrolimus are taken by renal transplant recipients for immunosuppression. These medications are metabolized by the cytochrome P450 system in the liver and thus, interact with a wide variety of agents. Care must be taken when starting or discontinuing any medication in a patient taking these agents, because the serum level may be affected. Diltiazem, statins, macrolides, and antifungal drugs inhibit the system, elevate levels, and can precipitate nephrotoxicity. Others, such as carbamazepine, barbiturates, and theophylline, induce the system, reduce levels, and can precipitate rejection. Drug levels must be monitored in this setting. IV cyclosporine and tacrolimus should be given at one-third the oral dose until the patient is able to tolerate oral medications. Of significant relevance to orthopedic surgery in which there may be concurrent use of warfarin and cyclosporine, these medications together can lead to decreased anticoagulant and cyclosporine effectiveness.[28] In such circumstances the levels of both warfarin and cyclosporine should be followed closely with dose adjustments made as needed. Any transplant patients taking chronic low-dose prednisone may require stress-dose steroids before surgery.

Lastly, patients on chronic immunosuppression are at increased risk for infections. Workup for the cause of fever should have a broader differential in the transplant patient. Those with a recent kidney transplant are at the highest risk. Should a transplant patient develop a life-threatening infection, the immunosuppressive agents may need to be held until the infection resolves, despite the risk of rejection and transplant failure.

SUMMARY

The prevalence of chronic and end-stage renal disease will continue to climb with the aging of the US population as well as increasing number of diabetics nationwide. In the setting of orthopedic surgery, many factors must be considered and appropriately assessed in the renal patient during the perioperative course. A multidisciplinary approach should be implemented during the assessment to reduce risk in regard to the patient's degree of renal insufficiency, need for renal replacement therapy, medications, anemia, and possible electrolyte imbalances. Although managing patients with renal disease can be challenging, careful preoperative evaluation and perioperative management can result in successful orthopedic surgical outcomes and reduce the risk of long-term renal complications following surgery.

REFERENCES

1. United States Renal Data System. CKD in the general population. 2015 USRDS annual data report: epidemiology of kidney disease in the United States [Chapter 1]. Bethesda (MD): National Institutes of Health, National Institute of Diabetes and Digestive and Kidney Diseases; 2015.
2. Xu GG, Yam A, Teoh LC, et al. Epidemiology and management of surgical upper limb infections in patients with end-stage renal failure. Ann Acad Med Singapore 2010;39(9):670–5.
3. Horio M, Orita Y, Fukunaga M. Assessment of renal function. Comprehensive clinical nephrology. Philadelphia: Mosby; 2000. p. 3.1–6.
4. National Kidney Foundation. K/DOQI clinical practice guidelines for chronic kidney disease: evaluation, classification, and stratification. Am J Kidney Dis 2002; 39(2 Suppl 1):3–4.
5. Anderson RJ, Schrier RW. Clinical spectrum of oliguric and non-oliguric acute renal failure. Contemporary Issues in Nephrology 1980;6:1–16.
6. Josephs SA, Thakar CV. Perioperative risk assessment, prevention and treatment of acute kidney injury. Int Anesthesiol Clin 2009;47(4):89–105.
7. Jafari SM, Huang R, Joshi A, et al. Renal impairment following total joint arthroplasty: who is at risk? J Arthroplasty 2010;25(Suppl 6):49–53.
8. Kheterpal S, Temper KK, Englesbe MJ, et al. Predictors of postoperative acute renal failure after noncardiac surgery in patients with previously normal renal function. Anesthesiology 2007;107(6):892–902.
9. Pavone V, Johnson T, Saulog PS, et al. Perioperative morbidity in bilateral one-stage total knee replacements. Clin Orthop Relat Res 2004;421:155–61.
10. Thakar CV, Arrigain S, Worley S, et al. A clinical score to predict acute renal failure after cardiac surgery. J Am Soc Nephrol 2005;16(1):162–8.
11. Wijeysundera DN, Karkouti K, Dupuis JY, et al. Derivation and validation of a simplified predictive index for renal replacement therapy after cardiac surgery. JAMA 2007;297(16):1801–9.
12. Kheterpal S, Tremper KK, Heung M, et al. Development and validation of an acute kidney injury risk index for patients undergoing general surgery: result from a national data set. Anesthesiology 2009;110(3):505–15.
13. Coriat P, Richer C, Douraki T, et al. Influence of chronic angiotensin-converting enzyme inhibition on anesthetic induction. Anesthesiology 1994;81(2):299–307.
14. Walker SS, Liu KD, Chertow GM. Diagnosis, epidemiology, and outcomes of acute kidney injury. Clin J Am Soc Nephrol 2008;3(3):844–61.
15. Kellerman PS. Perioperative care of the renal patient. Arch Intern Med 1994;154: 1674–88.
16. Craig RG, Hunter JM. Recent developments in the perioperative management of adult patients with chronic kidney disease. Br J Anaesth 2008;101(3):296–310.

17. Lee TH, Marcantonio ER, Mangione CM, et al. Derivation and prospective validation of a simple index for prediction of cardiac risk of major noncardiac surgery. Circulation 1999;100:1043–9.
18. Novis BK, Roizen MF, Aronson S, et al. Association of preoperative risk factors with postoperative acute renal failure. Anesth Analg 1994;78:143–9.
19. Lo LJ, Go AS, Chertow GM, et al. Dialysis-requiring acute renal failure increases the risk of progressive chronic kidney disease. Kidney Int 2009;76(8):893–9.
20. Hsu CY, Chertow GM, McCulloch CE, et al. Nonrecovery of kidney function and death after acute on chronic renal failure. Clin J Am Soc Nephrol 2009;4(5): 891–8.
21. Lafrance JP, Miller DR. Acute kidney injury associated with increased long-term mortality. J Am Soc Nephrol 2010;21(2):345–52.
22. Bennet SJ, Berry OM, Goddard J, et al. Acute renal dysfunction following hip fracture. Injury 2010;41(4):335–8.
23. Abelha FJ, Botelho M, Fernandes V, et al. Determinants of post-operative acute kidney injury. Crit Care 2009;13(3):R79.
24. London GM. Cardiovascular disease in chronic renal failure: pathophysiologic aspects. Semin Dial 2003;16:85–94.
25. Coresh J, Selvin E, Stevens LA, et al. Prevalence of chronic kidney disease in the United States. JAMA 2007;298(17):2038–47.
26. Brenowitz JB, Williams CD, Edwards WS. Major surgery in patients with chronic renal failure. Am J Surg 1977;134:765–9.
27. Schreiber S, Korzets A, Powsner E, et al. Surgery in chronic dialysis patients. Isr J Med Sci 1995;31:479–83.
28. Palevsky PM. Perioperative management of patients with chronic kidney disease or ESRD. Best Pract Res Clin Anaesthesiol 2004;18(1):129–44.
29. Kanda H, Hirasaki Y, Iida T, et al. Perioperative Management of patients with End-stage renal disease. J Cardiothorac Vasc Anesth 2017;31(6):2251–67.
30. Ahmed J, Weisberg LS. Hyperkalemia in dialysis patients. Semin Dial 2001; 14(5):348–56.
31. Kohagura K, Tomiyama N, Kinjo K, et al. Prevalence of anemia according to stage of CKD in a large screen cohort of Japanese. Clin Exp Nephrol 2009; 13(6):614–20.
32. Voormolen N, Grootendorst DC, Urlings TA, et al. Prevalence of anemia and its impact on mortality and hospitalization rate in predialysis patients. Nephron 2010;115(2):c133–41.
33. Karkouti K, Wijeysundera DN, Beattie WS. Reducing Bleeding in Cardiac surgery (RBC) investigators. Risk associated with preoperative anemia in cardiac surery: a multicenter cohort study. Circulation 2008;117(4):478–84.
34. De Santo L, Romano G, Della Corte A, et al. Preoperative anemia in patients undergoing coronary artery bypass surgery grafting predicts acute kidney injury. J Thorac Cardiovasc Surg 2009;138(4):965–70.
35. Beattie WS, Karkouti K, Wijeysundera DN, et al. Risk associated with perioperative eanemia in noncardiac surgery: a single-center cohort study. Anesthesiology 2009;110(3):574–81.
36. Mantilla CB, Wass CT, Goodrich KA, et al. Risk of perioperative myocardial infarction and mortality in patients undergoing hip or knee arthroplasty: the role of anemia. Transfusion 2011;51(1):82–91.
37. Kumar A. Perioperative management of anemia: limits of blood transfusion and alternatives to it. Cleve Clin J Med 2009;76(Suppl 4):S112–8.

38. Paganini EP. Hematologic abnormalities. In: Daugirdas JT, Ing TS, editors. Handbook of dialysis. 2nd edition. Boston: Little, Brown; 1994. p. 445–68.
39. Mannucci PM, Levi M. Prevention and treatment of major blood loss. N Engl J Med 2007;356(22):2301–11.
40. Lee HK, Kim YJ, Jeong JU, et al. Desmopressin improves platelet dysfunction measured by in vitro closure time in uremic patietns. Nephron 2010;114(4): c248–52.
41. Carless PA, Henry DA, MOxey AJ, et al. Desmopressin for minimising perioperative allogeneic blood transfusion. Cochrane Database Syst Rev 2004;(1). CDC001884.
42. Crescenzi G, Landoni G, Biondi-Zoccai G, et al. Demsopressin reduces transfusion needs after surgery: a meta-analysis of randomized controlled trials. Anesthesiology 2008;109(6):1063–76.
43. Chen KS, Huang CC, Leu ML, et al. Hemostatic and fibrinolytic response to desmopressin in uremic patients. Blood Purif 1997;15:84–91.
44. Davenport R. Cryoprecipitate for uremic bleeding. Clin Pharm 1991;10:429.
45. Steiner RW, Coggins C, Carvalho AC. Bleeding time in uremia: a useful test to assess clinical bleeding. Am J Hematol 1979;7:107–17.
46. Borthwick E, Ferguson A. Perioperative acute kidney injury: risk factors, recognition, management, and outcomes. BMJ 2010;341:85–91.
47. Bertrand M, Godet G, Meersschaert K, et al. Should the angiotensin II antagonists be discontinued before surgery? Anesth Analg 2001;92(1):26–30.
48. Rosenman DJ, McDonald FS, Ebbert JO, et al. Clinical consequences of withholding versus administering renin-angiotensin-aldosterone system antagonists in the perioperative period. J Hosp Med 2008;3(4):319–25.
49. Kheterpal S, Khodaparast O, Shanks A, et al. Chronic angiotensin-converting enzyme inhibitor or angiotensin receptor blocker therapy combined with diuretic therapy is associated with increased episodes of hypotension in noncardiac surgery. J Cardiothorac Vasc Anesth 2008;22(2):180–6.
50. Thakar CV, Kharat V, Blanck S, et al. Acute kidney injury after gastric bypass surgery. Clin J Am Soc Nephrol 2007;2(3):426–30.
51. Whinney C. Perioperative medication management: general principles and practical applications. Cleve Clin J Med 2009;76(Suppl 4):S126–32.
52. Rudnick M, Feldman H. Contrast-induced nephropathy: what are the true clinical consequences? Clin J Am Soc Nephrol 2008;3:263–72.
53. Maioli M, Toso A, Leoncini M, et al. Persistent renal damage after contrast-induced acute kidney injury: incidence, evolution, risk factors, and prognosis. Circulation 2012;125:3099–107.
54. Nemoto N, Iwasaki M, Nakanishi M, et al. Impact of continuous deterioration of kidney function 6 to 8 months after percutaneous coronary intervention for acute coronary syndrome. Am J Cardiol 2014;113:1647–51.
55. Droppa M, Desch S, Blase P, et al. Impact of N-acetylcysteine on contrast-induced nephropathy defined by cystatin C in patients with ST-elevation myocardial infarction undergoing primary angioplasty. Clin Res Cardiol 2011;100(11): 1037–43.
56. Ren L, Ji J, Fang Y, et al. Assessment of urinary N-Acetyl-ß-glucosaminidase as an early marker of contrast-induced nephropathy. J Int Med Res 2011;39(2): 647–53.
57. Briguori C, Visconti G, Rivera NV, et al. Cystatin C and contrast-induced acute kidney injury. Circulation 2010;121:2117–22.

58. Weisbord SD, Mor MK, Resnick AL, et al. Incidence and outcomes of contrast-induced AKI following computed tomography. Clin J Am Soc Nephrol 2008;3: 1274–81.

59. Barrett BJ, Katzberg RW, Thomsen HS, et al. Contrast-induced nephropathy in patients with chronic kidney disease undergoing computed tomography: a double-blind comparison of iodixanol and iopamidol. Invest Radiol 2006;41: 815–21.

60. Mitchell AM, Jones AE, Tumlin JA, et al. Incidence of contrast-induced nephropathy after contrast-enhanced computed tomography in the outpatient setting. Clin J Am Soc Nephrol 2010;5:4–9.

61. Solomon R. Contrast Media: are there differences in nephrotoxocity among contrast media? Biomed Res Int 2014;2014:934947.

62. Lautin EM, Freeman NJ, Schoenfeld AH, et al. Radiocontrast associated renal dysfunction: a comparison of lower-osmolality and conventional high-osmolality contrast media. AJR Am J Roentgenol 1991;157:59–65.

63. Kellum JA, Lamiere N, Aspelin P, et al. KDIGO. Clinical practice guideline for acute kidney injury. Kidney Int Suppl 2012;2:8.

64. Reed M, Meier P, Tamhane UU, et al. The relative renal safety of iodixanol compared with lowosmolar contrast media: a meta-analysis of randomized controlled trials. JACC Cardiovasc Interv 2009;2:645–54.

65. Eng J, Wilson RF, Subramaniam RM, et al. Comparative effect of contrast media type on the incidence of contrast-induced nephropathy: a systematic review and meta-analysis. Ann Intern Med 2016;164:417–24.

66. Persson PB, Hansell P, Liss P. Pathophysiology of contrast medium-induced nephropathy. Kidney Int 2005;68:14–22.

67. Zhang Y, Wang J, Yang X, et al. The serial effect of iodinated contrast media on renal hemodynamics and oxygenation as evaluated by ASL and BOLD MRI. Contrast Media Mol Imaging 2012;7:418–25.

68. Manske CL, Sprafka JM, Strony JT, et al. Contrast nephropathy in azotemic diabetic patients undergoing coronary angiography. Am J Med 1990;89:615–20.

69. Cigarroa RG, Lange RA, Williams RH, et al. Dosing of contrast material to prevent contrast nephropathy in patients with renal disease. Am J Med 1989;86: 649–52.

70. Zhang LJ, Qi L, Wang J, et al. Feasibility of prospectively ECG-triggered high-pitch coronary CT angiography with 30 mL iodinated contrast agent at 70 kVp: initial experience. Eur Radiol 2014;24:1537–46.

71. Chen CM, Chu SY, Hsu MY, et al. Low-tube-voltage (80 kVp) CT aortography using 320-row volume CT with adaptive iterative reconstruction: lower contrast medium and radiation dose. Eur Radiol 2014;24:460–8.

72. Szucs-Farkas Z, Schaller C, Bensler S, et al. Detection of pulmonary emboli with CT angiography at reduced radiation exposure and contrast material volume: comparison of 80 kVp and 120 kVp protocols in a matched cohort. Invest Radiol 2009;44:793–9.

73. Penfield JG, Reilly RF. What nephrologists need to know about gadolinium. Nat Clin Pract Nephrol 2007;3:654–68.

74. Fujisaki K, Ono-Fujisaki A, Kura-Nakamura N, et al. Rapid deterioration of renal insufficiency after magnetic resonance imaging with gadolinium-based contrast agent. Clin Nephrol 2011;75:251–4.

75. Perazella MA. Current status of gadolinium toxicity in patients with kidney disease. Clin J Am Soc Nephrol 2009;4:461–9.

76. Heinrich MC, Kuhlmann MK, Kohlbacher S, et al. Cytotoxicity of iodinated and gadolinium-based contrast agents in renal tubular cells at angiographic concentrations: in vitro study. Radiology 2007;242:425–34.

77. Saitoh T, Hayasaka K, Tanaka Y, et al. Dialyzability of gadodiamide in hemodialysis patients. Radiat Med 2006;24:445–51.

78. Parfrey PS, Griffiths SM, Barrett BJ, et al. Contrast material-induced renal failure in patients with diabetes mellitus, renal insufficiency, or both. A prospective controlled study. N Engl J Med 1989;320:143–9.

79. Mehran R, Aymong ED, Nikolsky E, et al. A simple risk score for prediction of contrast-induced nephropathy after percutaneous coronary intervention: development and initial validation. J Am Coll Cardiol 2004;44:1393–9.

80. Ranucci M, Castelvecchio S, Menicanti L, et al. Risk of assessing mortality risk in elective cardiac operations: age, creatinine, ejection fraction, and the law of parsimony. Circulation 2009;119:3053–61.

81. Capodanno D, Ministeri M, Dipasqua F, et al. Risk prediction of contrast-induced nephropathy by ACEF score in patients undergoing coronary catheterization. J Cardiovasc Med (Hagerstown) 2016;17:524–9.

82. Ozkok S, Ozkok A. Contrast-induced acute kidney injury: a review of practical points. World J Nephrol 2017;6(3):86–99.

83. Mueller C, Buerkle G, Buettner HJ, et al. Prevention of contrast mediaassociated nephropathy: randomized comparison of 2 hydration regimens in 1620 patients undergoing coronary angioplasty. Arch Intern Med 2002;162:329–36.

84. Trivedi HS, Moore H, Nasr S, et al. A randomized prospective trial to assess the role of saline hydration on the development of contrast nephrotoxicity. Nephron Clin Pract 2003;93:C29–34.

85. Nijssen EC, Rennenberg RJ, Nelemans PJ, et al. Prophylactic hydration to protect renal function from intravascular iodinated contrast material in patients at high risk of contrast-induced nephropathy (AMACING): a prospective, randomised, phase 3, controlled, openlabel, non-inferiority trial. Lancet 2017;389: 1312–22.

86. Brar SS, Aharonian V, Mansukhani P, et al. Haemodynamic-guided fluid administration for the prevention of contrast-induced acute kidney injury: the POSEIDON randomised controlled trial. Lancet 2014;383:1814–23.

87. Subramaniam RM, Suarez-Cuervo C, Wilson RF, et al. Effectiveness of prevention strategies for contrast-induced nephropathy: a systematic review and meta-analysis. Ann Intern Med 2016;164(6):406–16.

88. Kurella M, Bennett WM, Chertow GM. Analgesia in patients with ESRD: a review of available evidence. Am J Kidney Dis 2003;42(2):217–28.

89. Dean M. Opioids in renal failure and dialysis patients. J Pain Symptom Manage 2004;28(5):497–504.

90. Bailie GR, Mason NA. 2011 Dialysis of drugs. 2011th edition. Saline (MI): Renal Pharmacy Consultants, LLC; 2011.

91. Kursh ED, Klein L, Schmitt J, et al. The effect of uremia on wound tensile strength and collagen formation. J Surg Res 1977;23:37–42.

92. Shindo K, Kosaki G. Effects of chronic renal failure on wound healing in rats. II. Microscopic study and hydroxyproline assay. Jpn J Surg 1982;12:46–51.

93. Colin JF, Elliot P, Ellis H. The effect of uraemia upon wound healing: an experimental study. Br J Surg 1979;66:793–7.

94. Seth A, Garza M, Fang R, et al. Excisional wound healing is delayed in a Murine model of chronic kidney disease. PLos One 2013;8(3):1–10.

95. Yue DK, Swanson B. Abnormalities of granulation tissue and collagen formation in experimental diabetes, uraemia and malnutrition. Diabet Med 1986;3:221–5.
96. Turgeon NA, Perez S, Mondestin M. The impact of renal function on outcomes of bariatric surgery. J Am Soc Nephrol 2012;23:885–94.
97. Pollard J, Hamilton GA, Rush SM. Mortality and morbidity after transmetatarsal amputation: retrospective review of 101 cases. J Foot Ankle Surg 2006;45:91–7.
98. Azuma N, Uchida H, Kokubo T, et al. Factors influencing wound healing of critical ischaemic foot after bypass surgery: is the angiosome important in selecting bypass target artery? Eur J Vasc Endovasc Surg 2012;43:322–8.
99. Kawarada O, Yokoi Y, Higashimori A, et al. Impact of end-stage renal disease in patients with critical limb ischemia undergoing infrapopliteal intervention. EuroIntervention 2014;10:753–60.
100. Mahajan S. Zinc in kidney disease. J Am Coll Nutr 1989;8:296–304.
101. Thangarajah H, Yao D, Chang EI, et al. The molecular basis for impaired hypoxia-induced VEGF expression in diabetic tissues. Proc Natl Acad Sci U S A 2009;106:13505–10.
102. Vanholder R, Smet R, Glorieux G. Review on uremic toxins: classification, concentration, and interindividual variability. Kidney Int 2003;63:1934–43.
103. Baylis C. Nitric oxide synthase derangements and hypertension in kidney disease. Curr Opin Nephrol Hypertens 2012;21(1):1–6.
104. Wattanakit K, Folsom AR, Selvin E. Kidney function and risk of peripheral arterial disease: results from Atherosclerosis Risk in Communities (ARIC) Study. J Am Soc Nephrol 2007;18:629–36.
105. De Vinuesa SG, Ortega M. Subclinical peripheral arterial disease in patients with chronic kidney disease: prevalence and related risk factors. Kidney Int 2005;67: S44–7.
106. Rajagopalan S, Dellegrottaglie S. Peripheral arterial disease in patients with end-stage renal disease: observations from the Dialysis Outcomes and Practice Patterns Study (DOPPS). Circulation 2006;114:1914–22.
107. O'Hare AM. High prevalence of peripheral artery disease in persons with renal insufficiency: results from the National Health and Nutrition Examination Survey. Circulation 2004;109:320–3.
108. O'Hare A, Johansen K. Lower extremity peripheral arterial disease among patients with end-stage renal disease. J Am Soc Nephrol 2001;12:2838–47.
109. Ridker PM, Cushman M, Stampfer MJ. Plasma concentration of C-reactive protein and risk of developing peripheral vascular disease. Circulation 1998;97: 425–8.
110. Sethi D, Muller BR, Brown EA, et al. C-reactive protein in hemodialysis patients with dialysis arthropathy. Nephrol Dial Transplant 1988;3:269–71.
111. Hinchliffe RJ, Kirk B. The effect of hemodialysis on transcutaneous oxygen tension in patients with diabetes - a pilot study. Nephrol Dial Transplant 2006;21: 1981–3.
112. Fife CE, Buyukcakir C, Otto GH, et al. The predictive value of transcutaneous oxygen tension measurement in diabetic lower extremity ulcers treated with hyperbaric oxygen therapy: a retrospective analysis of 1144 patients. Wound Repair Regen 2002;10:198–207.
113. Kato S, Chimielewski M. Aspects of immune dysfunction in end stage renal disease. Clin J Am Soc Nephrol 2008;3:1526–33.
114. Cohen G, Haag-Weber M, Horl WH. Immune dysfunction in uremia. Kidney Int Suppl 1997;62:79–82.

115. Foley R. Infectious complications in chronic dialysis patients. Perit Dial Int 2008; 28(suppl 3):167–71.
116. Brodsky S, Nadasdy T, Rovin B, et al. Warfarin-related nephropathy occurs in patients with and without chronic kidney disease and is associated with an increased mortality rate. Kidney Int 2011;80(2):181–9.
117. Marckmann P. Nutritional status of patients on hemodialysis and peritoneal dialysis. Clin Nephrol 1988;29:75–8.
118. Daugirdas J, Blake P, Todd S. Handbook of dialysis. 4th edition. Lippincott Williams & Wilkins Publishers; 2007. p. 462–82.
119. Fouque D, Pelletier S, Mafra D, et al. Nutrition and chronic kidney disease. Kidney Int 2011;80:348–57.
120. Chertow GM, Goldstein-Fuchs DJ. Prealbumin, mortality, and cause-specific hospitalization in hemodialysis patients. Kidney Int 2005;68:2794–800.
121. Bansal VK, Vertuno LL. Surgery. In: Daugirdas JT, Ing TS, editors. Handbook of dialysis. 2nd edition. Boston: Little, Brown; 1994. p. 545–52.

Evaluation and Perioperative Management of the Diabetic Patient

Keith D. Cook, DPM[a],*, John Borzok, DPM[b], Fadwa Sumrein, DO[c], Douglas J. Opler, MD[d]

KEYWORDS

- Diabetes mellitus • Perioperative • Surgical complications • Diabetes management

KEY POINTS

- Patients with diabetes are at an overall higher risk of developing surgical complications.
- Surgical patients with diabetes need to be educated and well aware of the potential surgical outcomes and complications, and warrant a thorough preoperative evaluation including additional ancillary screening studies.
- Optimization of the patient's glucose levels before surgery when possible is ideal and may reduce the complications related to surgery in the patient with diabetes.
- Additional hardware, use of external fixation, prolonged immobilization, and non–weight bearing may be required in the patient with diabetes to enhance surgical outcomes.
- A multidisciplinary team approach to the perioperative management of the patient with diabetes should be used.

EVALUATION AND PERIOPERATIVE MANAGEMENT OF THE PATIENT WITH DIABETES

The podiatric surgeon can encounter many manifestations of the diabetic foot. Complications of the lower extremity may result secondarily from the diabetic process including ulcerations, infections, and Charcot neuroarthropathy. However, there are also patients with routine injuries and pedal pathology who coincidentally have diabetes and require special considerations during the perioperative period.

Diabetes is a chronic metabolic disorder characterized by hyperglycemia caused by impaired insulin production, insulin resistance, or a combination of both. According to

Disclosure Statements: Dr K.D. Cook is a consultant and speaker for DePuy Synthes and Osteomed. Drs J. Borzok, F. Sumrein, and D.J. Opler have no disclosures.
[a] Podiatry Department, University Hospital, 150 Bergen Street, Room G-142, Newark, NJ 07103, USA; [b] Podiatric Medicine and Surgery Residency Program, University Hospital, 150 Bergen Street, Room G-142, Newark, NJ 07103, USA; [c] Department of Medicine, Rutgers New Jersey Medical School, 185 South Orange Avenue, Newark, NJ 07103, USA; [d] Department of Psychiatry, Rutgers New Jersey Medical School, 185 South Orange Avenue, Newark, NJ 07103, USA
* Corresponding author.
E-mail address: cookkd@uhnj.org

Clin Podiatr Med Surg 36 (2019) 83–102
https://doi.org/10.1016/j.cpm.2018.08.004
0891-8422/19/© 2018 Elsevier Inc. All rights reserved.

the National Diabetes Statistical Report published by the Centers for Disease Control and Prevention in 2017, diabetes and prediabetes affects more than 100 million adults in the United States, with more than 9% of the population, about 30 million people, afflicted with diabetes in which 23 million are diagnosed and 7 million are undiagnosed.[1] According to the American Diabetes Association (ADA), in 2015, diabetes was the seventh leading cause of death in the United States, killing more Americans every year than AIDS and breast cancer combined. With the incidence increasing exponentially, it is considered a major public health epidemic.[1]

It is well documented that patients with diabetes have a greater risk of surgical complications than patients without diabetes. The perioperative management of these patients should be a multidisciplinary approach, using the experience and expertise of specialist and subspecialists to minimize or prevent complications and achieve successful results. The treatment care team may consist of foot and ankle surgeons, internists or hospitalists, endocrinologists, vascular surgeons, radiologists, nephrologists, cardiologists, psychiatrists, physical and occupational therapists, nutritionists, orthotists, and social workers to name a few.

A comprehensive history and physical examination along with appropriate ancillary studies are paramount in the preoperative period to assess for abnormalities and prevention of possible complications. The patient with diabetes requires medical optimization before bringing the patient to the operating room for any podiatric surgical procedure. This may consist of electrolyte balancing, lower extremity and/or cardiac revascularization, improved nutritional status, cessation of tobacco use, and improved glycemic control or kidney function. For those patients with end-stage renal disease elective surgical procedures should be planned around the patient's dialysis schedule. Postoperative care should also be planned in advance to determine if the patient can achieve and tolerate a non–weight bearing status if necessary or if in-patient rehabilitation services are required.

The anesthesiology team is also essential during this time, providing preoperative risk stratification for the patient and determining the safest mode of anesthesia and anesthetic agents to be used to prevent and limit intraoperative and postoperative complications. It is important the patient with diabetes understands the risks and complications associated with foot and ankle surgery. They must also understand that optimization must be continued throughout the perioperative period until complete healing and beyond. Surgery in patients with diabetes is linked to prolonged hospital stays, increases in perioperative morbidity and mortality, and rises in health care costs.[2] Therefore, awareness of perioperative needs and correct treatment protocols is vital to improving outcomes from many different vantage points.

UNDERSTANDING THE DIABETES MELLITUS PROCESS

Most diabetic cases are classified as type 1 or type 2 diabetes. Type 1 diabetics have impaired insulin production because of immune-mediated destruction of the pancreatic B islet cells, requiring insulin replacement.[3] The more prevalent type is type 2 diabetes. Type 2 diabetes is characterized as a relative insulin deficiency with many environmental and genetic factors playing a role in the cause.

Type 2 diabetes represents 80% to 90% of diabetes cases in the United States, usually presenting in adulthood. With an increasing obesity epidemic, type 2 diabetes is presenting at an earlier age. This is mostly caused by visceral obesity playing a large role in insulin resistance. There is a more insidious onset of hyperglycemia, usually asymptomatic. The elevated blood sugars are attributed to two main factors: tissue insensitivity to insulin and impaired β-cell compensation response to elevated blood sugars. The sustained hyperglycemia also effects insulin signaling and β-cell function. Over time, there is a β-cell functional decline, requiring insulin replacement in these patients.[4,5] Despite whether the patient is symptomatic or not, there are macrovascular and microvascular complications occurring, derived from the hyperglycemic state.

Because hyperglycemia is the key factor, it is used to make the diagnosis of diabetes or prediabetes. To further distinguish between type 1 and type 2 diabetes mellitus, antibodies are detected, such as glutamic acid decarboxylase 65, tyrosine phosphatase IA2, zinc transporter 8, and insulin auto antibodies.[6] Diagnosis of diabetes is determined by an elevated fasting blood sugar levels greater than or equal to 126 or a random glucose greater than 200 with symptoms, such as increase in urinary frequency, excessive thirst, or hunger. **Table 1** displays the plasma glucose and hemoglobin (Hb) A_{1C} ranges diagnostic criteria.[7] The 2-hour plasma glucose level is measured 2 hours after a 75-g load is given, to determine if the patient has an impaired response. More frequently HbA_{1C} values are used to determine diagnosis and further assess glycemic control in patients with diabetes. However, HbA_{1C} may not be accurate in patients with hemoglobinopathies, anemia, recent blood transfusions, uremia, and chronic liver disease.[8]

Diabetes increases the risk of a patient's morbidity and mortality. Acute life-threatening complications that can occur include hypoglycemia, coma, diabetic ketoacidosis, hyperglycemic hyperosmolar state, and lactic acidosis. Many of these conditions are characterized by severe volume depletion. This intravascular volume depletion predisposes patients to myocardial infarction, pulmonary embolism, and strokes. These complications can lead to death if not treated and managed without delay.

More commonly, chronic complications are the biggest detriment of patients with diabetes. Diabetes is considered an independent risk factor for cardiovascular disease. This is related to pathology at the microvascular and macrovascular levels. Macrovascular disease is described as a fast-tracked form of atherosclerosis; this predisposes patients to myocardial infarctions, strokes, and peripheral gangrene. Disease at the microvascular level is described as microvascular dysfunction and is attributed to a multitude of factors including "arteriovenous shunting, capillary leakage, precapillary sphincter malfunction, venous pooling, hormonal activity in the vessel, and inflammation in the vessel wall."[9] Also, increased protein glycation causes "stiffness" at the microvascular level. This microvascular dysfunction can lead to diabetic retinopathy, nephropathy, neuropathy, and can affect coronary arteries leading to coronary artery disease, and heart failure.[10–13]

Acute and chronic complications are reasonably controlled with appropriate glycemic control.[10] As demonstrated in **Table 2**, the Endocrine Society, ADA, and American Association of Clinical Endocrinologists (AACE) have set out glycemic

Table 1
Diagnostic criteria for diabetes

	Normal	Prediabetes	Diabetes
Fasting plasma glucose (mg/dL)	70–100	100–125	≥126
Hemoglobin A_{1c} (%)	<5.7	5.7–6.4	≥6.5
Plasma glucose 2 h after glucose load (mg/dL)	<140	140–199	≥200
Random glucose + symptomatic patient[a] (mg/dL)	—	—	>200

[a] Experiencing polyuria, polydipsia, or polyphagia.[7]

Modified from American Diabetes Association. Diagnosis and classification of diabetes mellitus. Diabetes Care 2010;33(Suppl 1):S62; with permission.

targets for adult patients.[14–17] These targets are adjusted for patients who are elderly, have multiple comorbidities, and/or critically ill patients. Management of patients with diabetes requires a comprehensive approach. Taking a detailed history and physical helps assess the presence of early complications. Treatment options vary depending on the type of diabetes. Patient education and self-management training is key in diabetes treatment regardless of the type. Type 1 diabetics require insulin replacement, with at least three-injection dosing. With new developments of continuous glucose monitoring and insulin pump systems, the management of hyperglycemia in treating type 1 diabetics has been simplified and the occurrence of treatment-related hypoglycemia has been minimized.[18,19] Type 2 diabetics have a more gradual progression of their disease. Treatment plans are based on level of β-cell function and insulin resistance. Patients are counseled on weight reduction; this includes caloric restriction and increased physical activity. In addition, patients are started on metformin. If a patient is unable to reach target glycemic targets, then other oral hypoglycemic agents are added, such as sulfonylureas, thiazolidinedione, alpha-glucosidase inhibitors, DDP-4 inhibitors, SGL2 inhibitors, and GLP-1 receptor agonist.[15–17,20–23] If patients fail improved glycemic control on oral therapy they are started on insulin therapy.

Approximately 25% of patients with diabetes require surgery, with an inherent increased risk of morbidity and mortality secondary to the presence of diabetes. Type 2 diabetes accounts for 16% of deaths from heart disease and stroke, 44% of end-stage renal failure, 60% of lower extremity amputation, and is associated with nonalcoholic fatty liver disease and polycystic ovarian syndrome.[24] Surgeries for these patients are usually high risk, again because of the microvascular and macrovascular disease. Therefore, all patients should be screened for diabetes preoperatively, because of the large incidence of unknown diabetics.

PREOPERATIVE EVALUATION: RISK STRATIFICATION AND COMORBIDITY AWARENESS

With respect to diabetes, goals for the perioperative management of these patients are to avoid hypoglycemia, avoid significant hyperglycemia, prevent ketoacidosis, and maintain fluid and electrolyte balance.[25] Achievement of these goals is predicated on a thorough preoperative history and physical examination. Obtaining specific information with respect to a patient's diabetic history, such as type of diabetes, history of diabetic complications, history of hypoglycemia, glycemic control, and current diabetic therapy, is essential to manage the diabetes perioperatively. Comorbidities must be identified, evaluated, and optimized.

The list of common diabetic comorbidities is expansive and includes but is not limited to obesity, dyslipidemia, hypertension, renal disease, cardiovascular disease, depression, sleep disorder, and many forms of cancer.[26] In a retrospective study, Suh and colleagues[27] investigated glycemic control among type 2 diabetics with potential comorbidities of hypertension, hyperlipidemia, and/or obesity. Only 14% of the

Table 2
Societal guidelines for glycemic control in adults

	ADA	AACE	Endocrine Society
Hemoglobin A_{1c}	<7.0	<6.5	—
Fasting	80–130	<110	<140
2 h post-prandial	<180	<140	<180

Data from Refs.[14–17]

type 2 diabetics did not have any additional comorbidity, whereas 21% had all three comorbidities. Given that comorbidities can develop within 6 years of diabetic diagnosis and many patients are unaware of diabetic diagnosis,[28] the evaluating physician should be prejudiced to the fact that every patient with diabetes has comorbidities until proven otherwise. Also, many of these comorbidities related to the diabetic surgical patient are a manifestation of the end-organ damage caused by chronic hyperglycemia.[28] The treating surgeon should be cognizant that this end organ damage can affect virtually any organ or system in the body. **Table 3** lists some of the diabetic-related damage throughout the body and attendant complications related to this damage. Because of the multitude of potential comorbidities and the overall complexity of this patient demographic, the preoperative evaluation of the diabetic surgical candidate should always involve the primary care physician and appropriate specialists.

In a review of 474 men undergoing noncardiac surgery, Hollenberg and colleagues[29] identified diabetes mellitus as an independent risk factor for developing postoperative myocardial ischemia. Cardiovascular pathology is the cause of death in 80% of patients with diabetes.[30] Because of the high prevalence of ischemic heart disease and that many patients with diabetes are asymptomatic, all patients with diabetes should have a recent electrocardiogram before surgery. Further evaluation via stress testing or other ancillary cardiac tests and examinations is at the discretion of primary care, cardiology, and/or anesthesiology. In most instances, the patient's primary care giver, internist, or family practice physician coordinates evaluations for these types of comorbidities. However, the foot and ankle physician should be aware of any eventuality with respect to comorbidities because the surgeon is involved with the patient's care from the beginning to completion. This is highlighted by the increasing use of hospitalists, where the preoperative evaluating physician often does not see the patient during hospitalization. In many instances, the foot and ankle surgeon is the only

Table 3
Diabetic complication and perioperative considerations

Complication	Perioperative Implication
Cardiovascular disease	

Myocardial ischemia/infarction
  Stroke
  Heart failure
	Major cause of perioperative morbidity and mortality

Autonomic neuropathy	
Cardiovascular	Risk of arrhythmia, consider telemetry
Cystopathy	Urinary retention, increased risk of UTI
Gastroparesis	Delayed gastric emptying, risk of reflux
Hypoglycemia unawareness	More frequent glucose monitoring
Nephropathy	Avoid IV contrast/nephrotoxic agents Appropriate hydration Monitor renal function
Peripheral neuropathy	Risk of skin breakdown, ulceration
Retinopathy	Can acutely worsen with blood loss
Cheiroarthropathy	Difficult intubation, positioning, and IV access
Impaired immunity/wound healing	Surgical site infection

Abbreviations: IV, intravenous; UTI, urinary tract infection.
Adapted from Miller JD, Richman DC. Preoperative evaluation of patients with diabetes mellitus. Anesthesiol Clin 2016;34:155–69; with permission.

provider who has any continuity of care and must be familiar with the patient's complete medical history and operative work-up.

Preoperative extremity vascular assessment initially focuses on the physical examination. It should be emphasized that both extremities should be evaluated and compared because this comparison can give subtle clues to different stages of vascular disease. Typical evaluation of skin turgor, digital/pedal hair growth and rubor on dependency, and pallor on evaluation should be performed on every patient, especially those with diabetes. The presence of pedal pulses and the absence of symptoms have a negative predictive value of 96% in excluding peripheral vascular disease in large vessels. However, the absence of pedal pulses has a sensitivity of 71% in predicting peripheral vascular disease, and dictates the need for further vascular assessment, including noninvasive vascular studies.[31] Indices of ankle/brachial pressure (ABI) are often unreliable in patients with diabetes as a result of the noncompressibility of calcified arteries, leading to false elevation of the index. More importantly, Bunte and colleagues[32] looked at the relationship between ABI and toe-brachial index and infragenicular arterial patency in patients with critical limb ischemia. Nearly one-third of the patients with any tissue loss (Rutherford 5 or 6) had a normal or mildly reduced ABI. This work was replicated in a separate study by Shishehbor and colleagues[33] where abnormal toe pressures in 24 cases of critical limb ischemia demonstrated normal ABI 29% of the time. ABI is a reflection of blood flow in the macrovasculature and does not reflect tissue perfusion, especially in those with diabetes. Other modalities, such as toe pressures, toe-brachial indices, and transcutaneous oxygen tension, are warranted to obtain a more accurate reflection of tissue perfusion and a potential proclivity for failure of wound healing.[34] Toe pressures have been shown to be more reliable, with healing of 85% at pressures greater than 45 mm Hg and of 36% between 30 mm Hg and 45 mm Hg. Transcutaneous oxygen tension greater than 30 mm Hg has a positive predictive value for healing of 90%. The equipment for measuring transcutaneous oxygen tension is expensive, and the testing is complex and time consuming.[35]

Other comorbidities that often complicate surgery in the patient with diabetes are renal disease and autonomic and peripheral neuropathy. Peripheral neuropathy is typically exhibited via pressure points and skin breakdown, which may lead to infection. But inherently, peripheral neuropathy represents increased chances of surgical site infection with diabetic foot and ankle surgery. Armstrong and colleagues[36] demonstrated a 6.7% infection rate in patients with diabetes who exhibited loss of protective sensation. In a series of articles, Wukich and colleagues[37–40] chronicled the presence of peripheral neuropathy as an independent risk factor for the development of postoperative surgical site infections. Specifically, the most recent article in this series, prospectively looked at 2060 foot and ankle surgeries performed by the same surgeon. In this article, patients with diabetes with complications exhibited neuropathy 97.3% of the time as demonstrated by a mean Michigan Neuropathy Screening Instrument score of 6.7 ± 2.1 (range, 0–10 and >2 considered as neuropathic). In these complicated patients with diabetes there was a factor increase of 7.25 with respect to surgical site infections compared with patients without diabetes without neuropathy and a 3.72-fold increase compared with uncomplicated patients with diabetes. Patients without diabetes with neuropathy had 4.72 factor increase rate of surgical site infections compared with patients without diabetes without neuropathy.[40] Domek and colleagues[41] demonstrated patients with diabetes with neuropathy had a 1.78 increased risk for developing a postoperative complication. In a retrospective study of 165 patients with diabetes undergoing osseous procedures,

Shibuya and colleagues[42] deduced peripheral neuropathy had the strongest association with bone healing complications.

Often much greater focus or appreciation is given to peripheral neuropathy as compared with autonomic neuropathy, especially by an extremity surgeon. However, autonomic neuropathy affects many organ systems throughout the body and inflicts significant morbidity as seen through the following manifestations: resting tachycardia, exercise intolerance, orthostatic hypotension, constipation, gastroparesis, sudomotor dysfunction, impaired neurovascular function, and hypoglycemic autonomic failure.[30] Clinically this may be seen as an increased risk and frequency for aspiration (acidity and content) or cardiac volatility associated with cardiac autonomic neuropathy (CAN) and an inability to increase heart rate, blood pressure, and cardiac output, especially after anesthetic induction.[43] CAN is also related to increased chances of cardiopulmonary arrest, hypothermia, silent myocardial ischemia, and ischemic strokes.[28] Up to 20% of patients with type 2 diabetes may suffer from CAN and this is most likely an underestimation because neuropathy and CAN are underappreciated.[43]

PREOPERATIVE EVALUATION: CAPACITY, CONSENT, AND PATIENT EXPECTATIONS

Behavioral and psychiatric considerations must also be included in perioperative management of the patient with diabetes. Before the procedure, informed consent should be sought by the primary provider by educating the patient on relevant medical information in nontechnical language. Such education should encompass the nature of the medical condition; the expected benefits of the recommended treatment; the risks involved; the inability to precisely predict outcome; the irreversibility of treatments; and the risks, benefits, and results or alternatives to no treatment. When attempts to obtain informed consent are stymied by patient factors, the patient's capacity to make decision may be in doubt. This may occur when the patient seems unable to understand the information presented, irrational around their decision making, unable to communicate a choice with a reasonable degree of consistency, or unable to appreciate that the situation actually applies and is not simply theoretic. Primary providers may assess capacity to proceed themselves when they are comfortable doing so, but in cases where capacity to make a medical decision is not obvious, expert opinion can be sought via psychiatric consultation.

Patient expectations around planned procedures should be elicited. Although optimism is helpful in motivating patients, the high likelihood of a future need for additional operative intervention may present the potential for future disappointment or even anger at the provider should the patient believe that procedures are definitive. Optimism can be productively encouraged by being realistically forthcoming with any potential for future rehabilitation and when necessary prosthetic placement. However, an unrealistically pessimistic or defeatist outlook on the part of a patient could preclude their willingness to proceed with care of treatable conditions. Overly negative predictions about the future are common in clinical depression and anxiety disorders and should prompt the clinician to screen the patient for the presence of these conditions, which themselves are potentially treatable. Again, expert opinion can be sought via psychiatric consultation.

PREOPERATIVE EVALUATION: GLYCEMIC CONTROL

The old adage, "the foot is attached to the rest of the body" is never more accurate than when a patient with diabetes is undergoing any foot or ankle surgical intervention. It is important to understand the potential surgical outcomes and complications associated with the patient with diabetes. In a review of diabetic ankle fractures, patients with chronic hyperglycemia had a 3.8-times higher risk of overall complications, 3.4-times higher noninfectious complications (malunion, nonunion, or Charcot neuroarthropathy), and five-times higher infectious complications compared with their uncomplicated diabetic counterparts.[39] Patients who maintain tighter glycemic control are also associated with fewer wound infections, shorter hospital stays, reductions in ischemia, and a lower mortality rate.[44] Because of this, glycemic maintenance should be assessed by measuring a HbA_{1c} preoperatively[45–48] to understand a patient's glycemic control and potentially to optimize before elective surgery. The risk of developing an infection or wound healing complications after elective, diabetic foot and ankle surgery goes up by a factor of 1.59 for every 1% increase in HbA_{1c}.[49] It should be noted that most investigation regarding preoperative HbA_{1c} and postoperative complications, specifically periarticular or deep infections, has been generated in a retrospective fashion evaluating total joint arthroplasty, specifically total knee arthroplasty. Two fundamental questions are at the forefront of these orthopedic investigations and, despite this narrow focus, the literature is clearly not definitive and may even be somewhat contentious. The two questions are as follows: in orthopedic surgery is there a linear relationship between HbA_{1c} and the propensity to develop a postoperative complication; and is there a threshold HbA_{1c} value where surgery higher than this number is prohibitive because of a precipitous increased complication rate?[50,51]

In 2017, Lopez and colleagues[50] reviewed literature to identify orthopedic studies that looked at preoperative HbA_{1c} and postoperative complications. This was done with emphasis placed on answering the previously stated questions in regards to preoperative HbA_{1c}; 13 studies met requirements and formed the main substance of this investigation.[52–64] Combining 5 of these 13 articles, they amassed a total of 83,848 patients with preoperative HbA_{1c} levels. Not one of these five papers concluded that elevated HbA_{1c} levels were related to increased rates of postoperative infection.[60–64] Specifically, Adams and colleagues[64] retrospectively looked 40,491 total knee replacements where 32,924 did not have diabetes, 5042 had controlled diabetes (HbA_{1c} <7.0%), and 2525 had uncontrolled diabetes (HbA_{1c} >7.0%). Demographics among the three groups were statistically deemed to have negligible differences and five specific complications were evaluated: (1) revision within 1 year, (2) deep infection within 1 year, (3) deep venous thromboses/pulmonary embolism within 90 days, (4) incident myocardial infarction within 1 year, and (5) all-cause hospitalization within 1 year. Just looking at the raw numbers with respect to deep infections may give some insight as to the relationship of HbA_{1c} levels and postoperative infections. The following infection rates were discovered: (1) nondiabetic, 216/32,924 (0.7%); (2) controlled diabetic, 58/5042 (1.2%); and (3) uncontrolled diabetic, 13/2525 (0.5%). Although not statistically significant, the uncontrolled diabetic group, with a mean HbA_{1c} of 7.6%, had just over one in five infections with half of the enrollees as compared with the controlled diabetics with a mean HbA_{1c} of 6.3%. One of the initial hypotheses of the authors on this paper was that patients with diabetes with a HbA_{1c} greater than 7.0% would be more likely to develop deep infections as compared with patients with diabetes with a HbA_{1c} less than 7.0%. None of the complications investigated demonstrated significant differences between any of the three groups and, most notably, total number of complications for the patients with controlled diabetes was 1877/5042 or 37% and for the patients with uncontrolled diabetes was 857/2525 or 34%.[64]

In the past 2 years Cancienne and colleagues[51,65–69] have retrospectively evaluated large, national databases to ascertain whether specific orthopedic procedures are at a greater risk of developing postoperative complications in patients with diabetes with an increasing HbA_{1c} and whether or not there is a threshold HbA_{1c}. They evaluated postoperative complications and perioperative HbA_{1c} in patients with diabetes undergoing open carpal tunnel release,[65] shoulder arthroplasty,[66] total hip arthroplasty,[67] total knee arthroplasty,[51] single level lumbar decompression,[68] and anterior cervical discectomy and fusion.[69] In all six reviews, the risk of postoperative complications increased as the HbA_{1c} increased.[51,64–69] This is counter to the paper of Lopez and colleagues.[50] Cancienne states that previous studies did not identify the relationship between HbA_{1c} and increased risk of postoperative complications because the number of patients with diabetes enrolled in these studies was too small.[51] With respect to identifying a specific HbA_{1c} threshold, the work of Cancienne is not consistent. The two spine papers identified a threshold of 7.5%,[68,69] the shoulder paper had a threshold of 8.0%,[66] and the open carpal tunnel paper had a threshold of 7% to 8%.[65] Neither the total knee nor total hip arthroplasty papers verified a threshold with an acceptable specificity and sensitivity.[51,67] The HbA_{1c} may not be a good "stand-alone" predictor of postoperative infection. The HbA_{1c} may not be an independent variable with a hard threshold number that may suggest precluding surgical risk. Other factors, such as body mass index, age, and other diabetic comorbidities, are contributory and should be included in this evaluation process.[50,51] With respect to the voluminous literature available concerning perioperative HbA_{1c} and potential postoperative complications, an answer of "yes" or "no" could be given to either one of the two questions posed at the beginning of this section. There is evidence to support either answer with each question.

There have been a few studies on diabetic foot and ankle surgery to evaluate the potential influence of perioperative HbA_{1c} levels and postoperative complications. There has been some concurrence in that investigators believe that as the HbA_{1c} goes up so does the complication rate.[30–37,42,70,71] The Wukich paper from 2014 is especially important because it is one of few, if not the only, prospective studies to evaluate perioperative HbA_{1c} and postoperative complications.[40] This study concluded that the risk of surgical site infection goes up when poor long-term glycemic control is encountered. Specifically, "multivariable logistic regression analysis demonstrated that peripheral neuropathy and a HbA_{1c} of greater than 8% were independently associated with surgical site infection."[40] One of the main differences in the foot and ankle papers is these authors investigated all diabetic foot and ankle surgeries and did not become entranced with the HbA_{1c} and its potential disturbance on any one, clean orthopedic procedure. Another issue that needs to be discussed more is that there is a tendency to want to compare coronary artery bypass grafting to total knee replacement to all foot and ankle surgery in patients with diabetes. At the very least the patient selection for these procedures is nowhere near the same and these are not true comparisons; and should not be formalized as such.

There is clearly a need for more prospective evaluation of the preoperative utility and appropriate threshold level of HbA_{1c}. Currently, recommendations continue to revolve around a HbA_{1c} of 7.0% as being a marker of the upper limit or "safe" level for surgery. It should be noted that the ADA originally used this HbA_{1c} level to signify the upper limit of acceptable glucose control to help avoid chronic complications associated with diabetes. This number has been assigned arbitrarily to preoperative risk stratification in surgical patients without scientific validation. MacKenzie and Gregory[25] recommend, in elective surgery, a HbA_{1c} of less than 7.0% represents satisfactory glucose control and levels greater than 10.0% represent levels that may merit cancellation of an elective surgical case. More importantly, recommendation for intermediate levels between 7.0% and 10.0% should be based on clinical judgment.[25] This is perhaps the most important statement of this section because the choice to cancel or proceed with a surgery should not be predicated solely by an HbA_{1c} number.

Such factors as length of surgery, invasiveness of procedure, history of present illness, need to improve functionality, and risks or repercussions of not having the surgery should all be factored into the overall decision. There is an assumption that canceling surgery and obtaining a better HbA_{1c} decreases the chances of experiencing postoperative complications. This assertion has not been studied. In many cases of extremity pathology, the proposition of a particular surgery has been made to improve function and activity level, such as a total knee replacement. Not moving forward with such a surgery may, in fact, perpetuate hyperglycemia by reducing activity and preventing positive lifestyle changes needed to reduce hyperglycemia.[50] In a more exaggerated example, seen in **Fig. 1**, this patient had a significant Charcot deformity and was nonambulatory for almost 6 months. All possible improvements were made with respect to comorbidities with the exception of the HbA_{1c}, which remained elevated at 8.3%. In this particular case, the patient underwent a successful, staged tibiocalcaneal arthrodesis. By no means does this suggest that the HbA_{1c} should be disregarded; it simply stresses that this and any other laboratory value should be placed in proper perspective.

PREOPERATIVE EVALUATION: DIABETIC PHARMACOLOGY

The most important component of handling diabetic medications in the perioperative period is proper communication between all treating physicians (surgeon, primary care physician, endocrinologist, and anesthesiologist) and appropriate education of the patient as to what changes and why these changes are being made with respect to diabetic medications perioperatively. It is important to try and make patients with diabetes the first surgeries of the day to minimize diabetic regimen changes and limit rate and severity of glycemic fluctuations. In general, oral hypoglycemic agents are held the

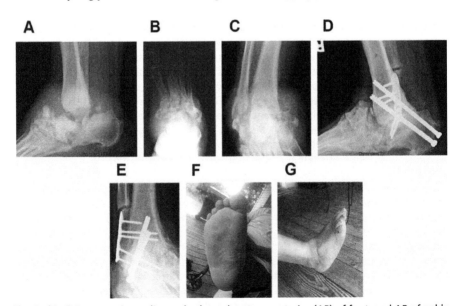

Fig. 1. (A–C) Preoperative radiographs: lateral, anteroposterior (AP) of foot, and AP of ankle. (D, E) Postoperative radiographs (30 weeks postoperative): lateral and AP ankle. (F, G) Clinical pictures 9 months postoperative.

day of surgery and not started until oral intake is resumed and tolerated. This is especially true of metformin. Recommendations are to hold this medication for 24 up to 48 hours preoperatively to avoid potential lactic acidosis. This is important to recognize because metformin is a cornerstone of many type 2 diabetes regimens. It is important to know some of the specifics of these medications, such as how they are metabolized. Many oral agents are metabolized by the kidney and it is essential to monitor and understand perioperative kidney function. If kidney function is transiently compromised with a long surgery and inadequate hydration, oral hypoglycemic agents started postoperatively may not be cleared as efficiently. This coupled with the typical decreased appetite after surgery may increase a patient's predisposition to develop hypoglycemia.

With respect to insulin and perioperative management the two tenets to keep in mind are the need to minimize hyperglycemia without risking a hypoglycemic episode.[72] With that in mind, it is important to make sure the patient knows to be aware of potential of hypoglycemic events and to have remedy on hand for any hypoglycemic symptoms. Patients should be instructed specifically that they are not to drive to the hospital when they are nothing by mouth status after taking a portion of long- or intermediate-acting insulin the night before or the morning of surgery. There should be protocol at the health care institution to process these patients quickly, start intravenous lines (IV), and obtain glucose readings as soon as the patient reaches preoperative area. It is preferable to keep the patient on the sweet side and titrate short-acting insulin accordingly than to cause hypoglycemia.

SURGERY AND PERIOPERATIVE GLUCOSE MANAGEMENT

Anesthesia and surgery is a form of trauma that causes a metabolic stress response for patients with and without diabetes.[73] However, in patients with preexisting glucose metabolism abnormalities, the release of catabolic hormones, such as epinephrine, cortisol, growth hormones, and glucagons, could overwhelm their homeostatic mechanisms.[74] This stimulation of gluconeogenesis and glycogenolysis inhibits insulin secretion and the effect is to essentially reverse the anabolic and anticatabolic actions of insulin, leading to potentially severe hyperglycemia.[74] To prevent escalation of the stress response in patients with diabetes, preoperative assessment of the patient should aim to optimize glycemic control before surgery. All medications should be evaluated by the patient's primary physician and anesthesia team before surgical intervention.

Surgery is a major stressor on the body, further impairing glycemic homeostasis (**Fig. 2**). Blood glucose levels need to be monitored carefully because they are unpredictable and difficult to control during this period.[75] Hyperglycemia is found in about 60% of patients who undergo cardiac surgery, regardless of their diabetes status.[76] It is associated with endothelial dysfunction; cerebral ischemia; postoperative sepsis; renal dysfunction; metabolic derangements; impaired wound healing; and in patients with diabetes, ketoacidosis and hyperglycemic hyperosmolar state.[76–78] The stress response is seen because of an increase in counterregulatory hormones, such as glucagon, corticosteroids, catecholamines, and growth hormone. These hormones lead to insulin resistance by inhibition of insulin release and impairing glucose uptake in peripheral tissues. There is also a stimulation of gluconeogenesis and glycogenolysis. Central nervous system involvement is also seen with increase in release of inflammatory cytokines that further promote insulin resistance and impaired endothelial function. Patients with diabetes who have impaired pancreatic function cannot compensate for the hyperglycemia.[79] Sufficient analgesia after surgery is essential in patients with diabetes because good pain relief reduces the metabolic responses and catabolic hormone secretion.[80]

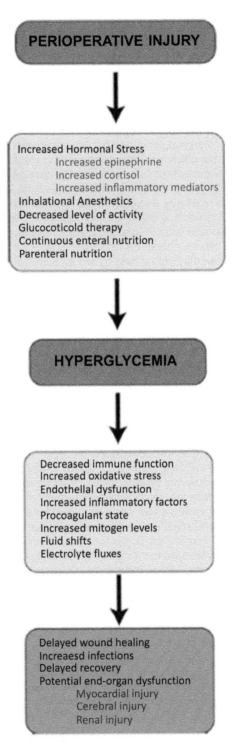

Fig. 2. Surgery and hyperglycemia. (*Adapted from* Attinger CE, Al-Attar A, Salgado C, et al. The importance of limb preservation in the diabetic population. J Diabetes Complications 2011;25(4):227–31; with permission.)

Although hyperglycemia should be avoided, hypoglycemia is also detrimental to the patient. Hypoglycemia is described as blood sugar less than 70. It is associated with high mortality and overall poor clinical outcomes. It also is associated with arrhythmias and increased cardiovascular events. Hypoglycemia may go unnoticed in patients who are critically ill or under anesthesia. Frequent glucose monitoring is important to ensure blood sugars do not fall too low. Dextrose solutions are used in the event a patient's blood sugar is not in the recommended ranges.[73,79] These factors contribute to the increase in morbidity associated with hyperglycemia and hypoglycemia. Many studies have been conducted to determine optimal blood glucose ranges to prevent complications and mortality. The overall consensus in the literature for patient with diabetes is blood sugar range between 140 mg/dL and 180 mg/dL. For stable patients without diabetes a blood sugar range can be lower between 110 mg/dL and 140 mg/dL.[77–79,81,82] Close monitoring of blood glucose, especially for unstable patients, should be every 1 to 2 hours. In the intensive care unit setting, this blood sugar range is usually achieved through IV insulin infusion, using standard nurse-driven protocols for titration. When patients are more hemodynamically stable and tolerating oral intake/nutritional support they are transitioned to subcutaneous insulin with 80% of IV insulin dose. Patients with diabetes are usually transitioned to basal-bolus insulin. For stable patients without diabetes, blood sugars are controlled with correction short-acting insulin. Sufficient analgesia after surgery is essential in patients with diabetes because good pain relief reduces the metabolic responses and catabolic hormone secretion.

SURGICAL TECHNIQUES IN THE PATIENT WITH DIABETES

Foot and ankle surgery in patients with diabetes has been linked to problems with soft tissue and bone healing. Therefore, patients with diabetes should be placed in a higher risk category for complications. Shibuya and colleagues[42] analyzed 165 patients with diabetes undergoing elective arthrodesis, reconstruction, or open reduction internal fixation of fractures. There was a statistically significant association for bone healing complication with peripheral neuropathy, surgery duration, and HbA_{1c} greater than 7%.

Because all patients with diabetes probably have some degree of microvascular dysfunction, proper tissue handling is imperative to prevent possible soft tissue damage and/or necrosis. Avoid or limit the use of self-retaining retractors because these can result in disruption of cutaneous blood supply and potentially increase incisional complications. Unnecessary grasping of cutaneous structures with forceps should be avoided. In addition, soft tissue healing is optimized when incisions are placed in accordance with the tenets of angiosomal blood distribution of the foot and ankle. Evans and colleagues[83] explained the angiosome concepts for the foot and ankle in great detail, with the safest incision bordering adjacent angiosomes. If an angiosome or its source artery is compromised from trauma or disease, then the incision should be placed within the ischemic angiosome territory to prevent damage to the patent angiosome.[83] When a staged surgical approach is mandated, such as trauma or infection cases, careful planning is imperative because the soft tissue envelope in the patient with diabetes, with comparatively marginalized blood flow, does not tolerate multiple, successive incisions if not placed or timed appropriately.

Frequent irrigation with or without antibiotics should be performed during surgery to help prevent wound desiccation and infection. During infected procedures surgical staff should exchange outer gloves and replace dirty instrumentation with sterile unused instruments after final irrigation to reduce cross-contamination.[84] Deep cultures and debrided tissue should be obtained intraoperatively in acutely infected surgical sites.

CONSIDERATIONS IN THE TRAUMA PATIENT WITH DIABETES

Unfortunately, optimization of the patient with diabetes is not always possible in the trauma or emergent setting. Soft tissue management is of paramount importance for any high-energy foot and ankle trauma and may be even more critical in patients with diabetes, who often have thin atrophic skin and impaired microcirculatory function. Prompt anatomic reduction of dislocations and application of a well-padded splint are crucial to decrease skin tension in a timely fashion. Nondisplaced fractures are typically treated nonoperatively with an increased duration of immobilization on average two times the period of patients without diabetes undergoing immobilization and non–weight bearing.[85]

Neuropathic fractures have been the subject of much research in the past decade. In one study, diabetic ankle fractures that were treated surgically had an overall complication rate of 14%.[85] It is well accepted these fractures require additional fixation and an extended non–weight bearing status for these patients (**Fig. 3**). Neuropathic fractures are prone to developing Charcot neuroarthropathy and close postoperative follow-up with serial radiographs to evaluate healing is required. The use of locking plates in this patient population with poor bone quality is advantageous over nonlocking plate technology. The locked screws rely on the plate as opposed to the bone to achieve fixation and a stable construct to allow for bone healing. Reduced disruption of the soft tissue envelope and periosteal vascular supply can also be achieved via minimally invasive percutaneous osteosynthesis techniques.

In the poly-traumatized patient, those with compromised lower extremity vascular supply, or a poor soft tissue envelope, definitive fracture fixation may not be achievable

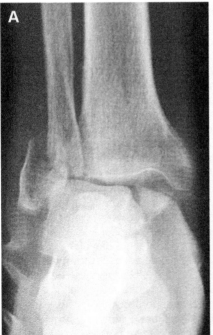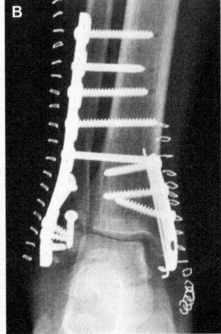

Fig. 3. (A) Patient with diabetes with neuropathy who sustained displaced bimalleolar ankle fracture. (B) Fixation was achieved with additional fixation and multiple transsyndesmotic screws.

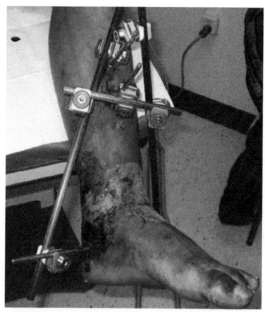

Fig. 4. Patient with diabetes with soft tissue compromise and an unstable left ankle fracture. A Delta frame was used to stabilize the fractures, allowing for the soft tissue envelope to heal before conversion to internal fixation.

at the initial operative setting. The use of external fixation for stabilization of these fractures should be considered in staging these patients until internal fixation can be used. In many cases a simple Delta frame construct can produce the desirable results (**Fig. 4**).

SUMMARY

Patients with diabetes with chronic, poorly controlled hyperglycemia are estimated to be four times higher risk of developing overall surgical complications when compared with patients with tighter glycemic control. These complications can be minor forms of morbidity, such as prolonged wound healing; significant morbidity, such as deep infection and below knee amputation; or even mortality. Because of this wide spectrum and potentially catastrophic outcomes, it is important to implement a multidisciplinary approach to the perioperative evaluation and management of this patient demographic. This approach allows for the requisite evaluation of this multifaceted pathology. It should be emphasized that the foot and ankle specialist should be aware of not only the local manifestations of this disease process but also the wide-ranging systemic consequences of diabetes. This includes the behavioral and psychiatric consequences of the diabetic process.

REFERENCES

1. Centers for Disease Control and Prevention. National diabetes statistics report, 2017. Atlanta (GA): Centers for Disease Control and Prevention, U.S. Dept. of Health and Human Services; 2017.
2. C Holt P. Pre and post-operative needs of patients with diabetes. Nurs Stand 2012;26(50):50–6.

3. Chiang JL, Kirkman MS, Laffel LM, et al. Type 1 diabetes through the life span: a position statement of the American Diabetes Association. Diabetes Care 2014;37: 2034.

4. Sullivan PW, Morrato EH, Ghushchyan V, et al. Obesity, inactivity, and the prevalence of diabetes and diabetes-related cardiovascular comorbidities in the U.S., 2000-2002. Diabetes Care 2005;28:1599.

5. Stumvoll M, Goldstein BJ, van Haeften TW. Type 2 diabetes: principles of pathogenesis and therapy. Lancet 2005;365:1333.

6. Bluestone JA, Herold K, Eisenbarth G. Genetics, pathogenesis and clinical interventions in type 1 diabetes. Nature 2010;464:1293.

7. American Diabetes Association. Diagnosis and classification of diabetes mellitus. Diabetes Care 2010;33(Suppl 1):S62.

8. Radin MS. Pitfalls in hemoglobin A1c measurement: when results may be misleading. J Gen Intern Med 2014;29(2):388–94.

9. Nouvong A, Armstrong DG. Diabetic foot ulcers. In: Cronenwett JL, Johnston KW, editors. Rutherford's vascular srugery. 8th edition. Philadelphia: Elsevier; 2014 [Chapter 116].

10. The Diabetes Control and Complications Trial Research Group. The effect of intensive treatment of diabetes on the development and progression of long-term complications in insulin-dependent diabetes mellitus. N Engl J Med 1993; 329:977–86.

11. Klein R, Klein BE, Moss SE, et al. Relationship of hyperglycemia to the long-term incidence and progression of diabetic retinopathy. Arch Intern Med 1994;154: 2169.

12. Bash LD, Selvin E, Steffes M, et al. Poor glycemic control in diabetes and the risk of incident chronic kidney disease even in the absence of albuminuria and retinopathy: atherosclerosis Risk in Communities (ARIC) Study. Arch Intern Med 2008;168:2440.

13. ADVANCE Collaborative Group, Patel A, MacMahon S, Chalmers J, et al. Intensive blood glucose control and vascular outcomes in patients with type 2 diabetes. N Engl J Med 2008;358:2560.

14. American Diabetes Association. 2. Classification and diagnosis of diabetes. Diabetes Care 2017;40:S11.

15. Garber AJ, Abrahamson MJ, Barzilay JI, et al. Consensus statement by the American Association of Clinical Endocrinologists and American College of Endocrinology on the comprehensive type 2 diabetes management algorithm: 2017 executive summary. Endocr Pract 2017;23(1):207–38.

16. Handelsman Y, Bloomgarden ZT, Grunberger G, et al. American Association of Clinical Endocrinologists and American College of Endocrinology: clinical practice guidelines for developing a diabetes mellitus comprehensive care plan– 2015. Endocr Pract 2015;21(0):1–87.

17. American Diabetes Association. 6. Glycemic targets. Diabetes Care 2017;40(Suppl 1):S48–56.

18. Nathan DM, Cleary PA, Backlund JY, et al. Intensive diabetes treatment and cardiovascular disease in patients with type 1 diabetes. N Engl J Med 2005;353: 2643.

19. Grunberger G, Handelsman Y, Bloomgarden ZT, et al. American Association of Clinical Endocrinologists and American College of Endocrinology 2018 position statement on integration of insulin pumps and continuous glucose monitoring in patients with diabetes mellitus. Endocr Pract 2018;24(3):302–8.

20. American Diabetes Association. Standards of medical care in diabetes -2018. Diabetes care, American Diabetes Association. 2018. Available at: care. diabetesjournals.org/content/41/Supplement_1/S7.
21. American Diabetes Association. 3. Comprehensive medical evaluation and assessment of comorbidities. Diabetes Care 2017;40:S25.
22. Nathan DM, Buse JB, Davidson MB, et al. Management of hyperglycemia in type 2 diabetes: a consensus algorithm for the initiation and adjustment of therapy: a consensus statement from the American Diabetes Association and the European Association for the Study of Diabetes. Diabetes Care 2006;29:1963.
23. Nathan DM, Buse JB, Davidson MB, et al. Medical management of hyperglycemia in type 2 diabetes: a consensus algorithm for the initiation and adjustment of therapy: a consensus statement of the American Diabetes Association and the European Association for the Study of Diabetes. Diabetes Care 2009;32:193.
24. Nolan CJ, Damm P, Prentki M. Type 2 diabetes across generations: from pathophysiology to prevention and management. Lancet 2011;378(9786):169–81.
25. Mackenzie CR, Gregory NS. Perioperative care of the orthopedic patient with diabetes mellitus. In: Mackenzie CR, Cornell CN, Memtsoudis SG, editors. Perioperative care of the orthopedic patient. New York: Springer; 2014 [Chapter 14].
26. AACE diabetes resource center. Available at: http://outpatient.aace.com/type-2-diabetes/management-of-common-comorbidities-of-diabetes.
27. Suh DC, Choi IS, Plauschinat C, et al. Impact of comorbid conditions and race/ethnicity on glycemic control among the US population with type 2 diabetes, 1988-1994 to 1999-2004. J Diabetes Complications 2010;24:382–91.
28. Miller JD, Richman DC. Preoperative evaluation of patients with diabetes mellitus. Anesthesiol Clin 2016;34:155–69.
29. Hollenberg M, Mangano DT, Browner WS, et al. Predictors of postoperative myocardial ischemia in patients undergoing noncardiac surgery. The study of perioperative ischemia research group. JAMA 1992;268(2):205–9.
30. Kadoi Y. Anesthetic considerations in the diabetic patient. Part 1: preoperative considerations of patients with diabetes mellitus. J Anesth 2010;24:739–47.
31. Criqui MH, Fronek A, Klauber MR, et al. The sensitivity, specificity, and predictive value of traditional clinical evaluation of peripheral arterial disease: results from noninvasive testing in a defined population. Circulation 1985;71:516–22.
32. Bunte MC, Jacob J, Nudelman B, et al. Validation of the relationship between ankle-brachial and toe-brachial indices and infragenicular arterial patency in critical limb ischemia. Vasc Med 2015;1:23–9.
33. Shishehbor MH, Hammad TA, Zeller T, et al. An analysis of IN.PACT DEEP randomized trial on the limitations of the societal guidelines-recommended hemodynamic parameters to diagnose critical limb ischemia. J Vasc Surg 2016;63(5):1311–7.
34. Stone PA, Glomski A, Thompson SN, et al. Toe pressures are superior to duplex parameters in predicting wound healing following toe and foot amputations. Ann Vasc Surg 2018;46:147–54.
35. Kalani M, Brismar K, Fagrell B, et al. Transcutaneous oxygen tension and toe blood pressure as predictors for outcome of diabetic foot ulcers. Diabetes Care 1999;22:147–51.
36. Armstrong DG, Lavery LA, Frykberg RG, et al. Validation of a diabetic foot surgery classification. Int Wound J 2006;3:240–6.
37. Wukich DK, Lowery NJ, McMillen RL, et al. Postoperative infection rates in foot and ankle surgery: a comparison of patients with and without diabetes mellitus. J Bone Joint Surg Am 2010;92:287.

38. Wukich DK, McMillen RL, Lowery NJ, et al. Surgical site infections after foot and ankle surgery: a comparison of patients with and without diabetes. Diabetes Care 2011;34:2211.

39. Wukich DK, Joseph A, Ryan M, et al. Outcomes of ankle fractures in patients with uncomplicated versus complicated diabetes. Foot Ankle Int 2011;32(2):120–30.

40. Wukich DK, Crim BE, Frykberg RG, et al. Neuropathy and poorly controlled diabetes increases the rate of surgical site infection after foot and ankle surgery. J Bone Joint Surg Am 2014;96(10):832–9.

41. Domek N, Dux K, Pinzur M, et al. Association between hemoglobin a1c and surgical morbidity in elective foot and ankle surgery. J Foot Ankle Surg 2016;55: 939–43.

42. Shibuya N, Humphers JM, Fluhman BL, et al. Factors associated with nonunion, delayed union, and malunion if foot and ankle surgery in diabetic patients. J Foot Ankle Surg 2013;52(2):207–11.

43. Vinik AI. Diabetic autonomic neuropathy. Diabetes Care 2003;26:1553–79.

44. Burns P, Highlander P, Shinabarger A. Management in high-risk patients. Clin Podiatr Med Surg 2014;31:523–38.

45. Dhatariya K, Levy N, Kilvert A, et al. NHS diabetes guidelines for the perioperative management of the adult patient with diabetes. Diabetic Med 2012;29(4): 420–3.

46. Jacober SJ, Sowers JR. An update on perioperative management of diabetes. Arch Intern Med 1999;159:2405.

47. Schricker T, Gougeon R, Eberhart L, et al. Type 2 diabetes mellitus and the catabolic response to surgery. Anesthesiology 2005;102:320.

48. Gavin LA. Perioperative management of the diabetic patient. Endocrinol Metab Clin North Am 1992;21:457.

49. Humpfers JM, Shibuya N, Fluhman BL, et al. The impact of glycosylated hemoglobin on wound-healing complications and infection after foot and ankle surgery. J Am Podiatr Med Assoc 2014;104(4):370–9.

50. Lopez LF, Reaven PD, Harman SM. Review: the relationship of HbA1c to postoperative surgical risk with an emphasis on joint replacement surgery. J Diabetes Complications 2017;31:1710–8.

51. Cancienne JM, Werner BC, Browne JA, et al. Is there an association between hemoglobin A1C and deep postoperative infection after TKA? Clin Orthop Relat Res 2017;475:1642–9.

52. Hwang JS, Kim SJ, Bamne AB, et al. Do glycemic markers predict occurrence of complications after total knee arthroplasty in patients with diabetes? Clin Orthop Relat Res 2015;473(5):1726–31.

53. Jamsen E, Nevalainen P, Kalliovalkama J, et al. Preoperative hyperglycemia predicts infected total knee replacement. Eur J Intern Med 2010;21(3):196–201.

54. Stryker LS, Abdel M, MorreyME, et al. Elevated postoperative blood glucose and preoperative hemoglobin A1C are associated with increased wound complications following total joint arthroplasty. J Bone Joint Surg Am 2013;95(9):808–14 [S1-2].

55. Moon HK, Han CD, Yang IH, et al. Factors affecting outcome after total knee arthroplasty in patients with diabetes mellitus. Yonsei Med J 2008;49(1):129–37.

56. Iorio R, Williams KM, Marcantonio AJ, et al. Diabetes mellitus, hemoglobin A1C, and the incidence of total joint arthroplasty infection. J Arthroplasty 2012;27(5): 726–9 [e1].

57. Lamloum SM, Mobasher LA, Karar AH, et al. Relationship between postoperative infectious complications and glycemic control for diabetic patients in an orthopedic hospital in Kuwait. Med Princ Pract 2009;18(6):447–52.

58. Goldstein DT, Durinka JB, Martino N, et al. Effect of preoperative hemoglobin A(1c) level on acute postoperative complications of total joint arthroplasty. Am J Orthop (Belle Mead NJ) 2013;42(10):E88–90.

59. Han HS, Kang SB. Relations between long-term glycemic control and postoperative wound and infectious complications after total knee arthroplasty in type 2 diabetics. Clin Orthop Surg 2013;5:118–23.

60. Chrastil J, Anderson MB, Stevens V, et al. Is hemoglobin A1c or perioperative hyperglycemia predictive of periprosthetic joint infection or death following primary total joint arthroplasty? J Arthroplasty 2015;30(7):1197–202.

61. Harris AH, Bowe TR, Gupta S, et al. Hemoglobin A1C as a marker for surgical risk in diabetic patients undergoing total joint arthroplasty. J Arthroplasty 2013;28(8 Suppl):25–9.

62. King JT, Goulet JL, Perkal MF, et al. Glycemic control and infections in patients with diabetes undergoing noncardiac surgery. Ann Surg 2011;253(1):158–65.

63. Kremers HM, Lewallen L, Mabry TM, et al. Diabetes mellitus, hyperglycemia, hemoglobin A1c and the risk of prosthetic joint infections in total hip and knee arthroplasty. J Arthroplasty 2015;30(3):439–43.

64. Adams AL, Paxton EW, Wang JQ, et al. Surgical outcomes of total knee replacement according to diabetes status and glycemic control, 2001 to 2009. J Bone Joint Surg Am 2013;95(6):481–7.

65. Werner BC, Teran VA, Cancienne J, et al. The association of perioperative glycemic control with postoperative surgical site infection following open carpal tunnel release surgery. Hand (N Y) 2017. [Epub ahead of print].

66. Cancienne J, Breckmeier SF, Werner BC. Association of perioperative glycemic control with deep postoperative infection after shoulder arthroplasty in patients with diabetes. J Am Acad Orthop Surg 2018;26(11):e238–45.

67. Cancienne JM, Werner BC, Browne JA. Is there a threshold value of hemoglobin A1c that predicts risk of infection following primary total hip arthroplasty? J Arthroplasty 2017;32(9s):s234–40.

68. Cancienne JM, Werner BC, Chen DQ, et al. Perioperative hemoglobin A1c as a predictor of deep infection following single-level lumbar decompression in patients with diabetes. Spine J 2017;17(8):1100–5.

69. Cancienne JM, Werner BC, Hassanzadeh H, et al. The association of perioperative glycemic control with deep postoperative infection after anterior cervical discectomy and fusion in patients with diabetes. World Neurosurg 2017;102:13–7.

70. Jupiter DC, Humphers JM, Shibuya N. Trends in postoperative infection rates and their relationship to glycosylated hemoglobin levels in diabetic patients undergoing foot and ankle surgery. J Foot Ankle Surg 2014;53(3):307–11.

71. Myers TG, Lowery NJ, Frykberg RG, et al. Ankle and hindfoot fusions: comparison of outcomes in patients with and without diabetes. Foot Ankle Int 2012;33:20.

72. Cornelius BW. Patients with type 2 diabetes: anesthetic management in the ambulatory setting: part 2: pharmacology and guidelines for perioperative management. Anesth Prog 2017;64:39–44.

73. Sudhakaran S, Salim RS. "Guidelines for perioperative management of the diabetic patient." Surgery research and practice. Cairo (Egypt): Hindawi; 2015. Available at: www.hindawi.com/journals/srp/2015/284063/.

74. Ramos M, Khalpey Z, Lipsitz S, et al. Relationship of perioperative hyperglycemia and postoperative infections in patients who undergo general and vascular surgery. Ann Surg 2008;248(4):585–91.

75. National Health Service 2011 management of adults with diabetes undergoing surgery and elective procedures: improving standards. Available at: https://www.diabetes.org.uk.

76. Mendez CE, Mok KT, Ata A, et al. Increased glycemic variability is independently associated with length of stay and mortality in non-critically ill hospitalized patients. Diabetes Care 2013;36(12):4091–7.

77. Ascione R, Rogers CA, Rajakaruna C, et al. Inadequate blood glucose control is associated with in-hospital mortality and morbidity in diabetic and nondiabetic patients undergoing cardiac surgery. Circulation 2008;118(2):113–23.

78. Falciglia M, Freyberg RW, Almenoff PL, et al. Hyperglycemia-related mortality in critically ill patients varies with admission diagnosis. Crit Care Med 2009;37(12): 3001–9.

79. Galindo R, Fayfman M, Umpierrez G. Perioperative management of hyperglycemia and diabetes in cardiac surgery patients. Endocrine and metabolism clinic. 2018. Available at: http://www.endo.theclinics.com/article/S0889-8529(17)30101-9/pdf. Accessed March 1, 2018.

80. Kaynes MN, Prodham NM, Malik RH. Perioperative management of diabetes: a review. Delta Medical College Journal 2014;2(2):71–6.

81. Frisch A, Chandra P, Smiley D, et al. Prevalence and clinical outcome of hyperglycemia in the perioperative period in noncardiac surgery. Diabetes Care 2010;33(8):1783–8.

82. Carvalho G, Moore A, Qizilbash B, et al. Maintenance of normoglycemia during cardiac surgery. Anesth Analg 2004;99(2):319–24.

83. Evans KK, Attinger CE, Al-Attar A, et al. The importance of limb preservation in the diabetic population. J Diabetes Complications 2011;25(4):227–31.

84. Roukis T. Bacterial skin contamination before and after surgical preparation of the foot, ankle, and lower leg in patients with diabetes and intact skin versus patients with diabetes and ulceration: a prospective controlled therapeutic study. J Foot Ankle Surg 2010;49:348–56.

85. Bibbo C, Lin SS, Beam HA, et al. Complications of ankle fractures in diabetic patients. Orthop Clin North Am 2001;32(1):113–33.

Perioperative Cardiac Considerations in the Surgical Patient

Rameez Sayyed, MD, FSCAI, Mian Bilal Alam, MD*

KEYWORDS

- Coronary artery disease • Risk factors • Risk stratification • Metabolic equivalencies
- Cardiology consultation • Revised Cardiac Risk Index • Defibrillator
- Medication recommendations

KEY POINTS

- Cardiology consultation is advisable in foot and ankle surgical candidates with cardiac history.
- Understanding cardiac risk allows for appropriate risk stratification.
- Appropriate risk stratification involves patient-, surgeon-, and procedure-related factors.
- Appreciation for assessment of functional capacity assists in delineating patients at higher risk for major adverse cardiac events in the perioperative time frame.
- With an aging population, more and more instances will require basic understanding of management principles regarding cardiovascular implantable electronic devices.

Worldwide volume of surgery is large and in view of the high death and complication rates associated with major surgical procedures, surgical safety should be a substantial global public health concern. Annually, 1 in every 40 adults has a major noncardiac surgery, which is defined as surgery requiring an overnight hospital admission.[1] More than 10 million of the 200 million patients having surgery suffer a major cardiac complication (eg, cardiac death, myocardial injury, cardiac arrest) in the first month after surgery.[2] Perioperative cardiac complications hence are critical because they account for at least one-third of perioperative deaths. They result in considerable morbidity and prolonged hospitalization[3] along with an increased cost,[4] and affect intermediate- and long-term prognosis. Because of this, often patients considered for foot and ankle surgery with a history of cardiac disease or signs and symptoms suggestive of cardiac disease should have cardiac evaluation. Some situations do not allow for this, such as

Disclosure Statements: None.
Department of Adult Cardiovascular Medicine, Joan C. Edwards School of Medicine, Marshall University, 1249 15th Street, Suite 4000, Huntington, WV 25701, USA
* Corresponding author.
E-mail address: alamm@marshall.edu

emergency surgery, and some situations may not require this, such as minor surgery under local anesthesia with sedation (eg, a fifth digital arthroplasty). However, in every surgical candidate, open dialogue between primary care physician, anesthesiologist, and surgeon helps develop consensus in regards to cardiology involvement. This consensus is formulated on patient characteristics, type of anesthesia required, and severity of surgery. It is extremely uncommon to regret obtaining a cardiology consultation; however, the corollary is not true because many perioperative major adverse cardiac events (MACE) potentially could be eliminated or lessened with preoperative cardiology participation.

The first and primary focus of the preoperative cardiac evaluation is to assess the risk of a cardiac event perioperatively. Once risk assessment has been determined, attention is then focused on any interventions that can be administered or performed to minimize risk and optimize cardiac function perioperatively. In discussing a cardiology consultation with a given patient it should be emphasized to the patient that this action is being taken to evaluate and optimize from a cardiac standpoint. Referring surgeons and any health care provider involved with perioperative evaluation and treatment of a patient should refrain from using the term "clearance" because this gives the wrong connotation that there will be no problems with a proposed surgical intervention once "clearance" is obtained. A discussion should take place with the patient to convey concerns about established or potential cardiac disease and attendant risks and how to minimize these risks related to surgery. The patient should be specifically told that even though several steps may be taken to avoid a perioperative cardiac event, a cardiac problem could still occur and the entire process is part of the risk/benefit decision process undertaken for any surgical intervention.

Because of the high rate of mortality associated with perioperative myocardial infarction (MI) coupled with the fact that patients with a history of MI or signs and symptoms associated with cardiac disease have increased predilection for perioperative MI, risk stratification for cardiac disease has evolved.[5] Originally, Goldman developed a multifactorial system for the assessment of cardiac disease after multivariate analysis of nine clinical and historical features in 1001 patients undergoing noncardiac surgery. This cardiac risk stratification was based on the following parameters: (1) history: age greater than 70 (5 points) and history of MI within 6 months (10 points); (2) cardiac examination: signs of congestive heart failure (ventricular gallop or jugular venous distention; 11 points) and significant aortic stenosis (3 points); (3) electrocardiograph: arrhythmia other than sinus or premature atrial contracture (7 points) and five or more premature ventricular contractions per minute (7 points); (4) general medical condition: Po_2 less than 60, Pco_2 less than 50, potassium less than 3, HCO_3 less than 20, blood urea nitrogen greater than 50, creatinine greater than three, elevated serum glutamic oxaloacetic transaminase, chronic liver disease, or bedridden (3 points); and (5) operation: emergency (4 points) and intraperitoneal, intrathoracic, or aortic (3 points). The following classes and correlative risk were established after adding points allocated for the previously mentioned parameters: 0 to 5 points, class I, 1% complications; 6 to 12 points, class II, 7% complications; 13 to 25 points, class III, 14% complications; and 26 to 53 points, class IV, 78% complications. This system was designed not only to identify risk factors but also to delineate reversible cardiovascular factors that could be improved on or corrected before surgery.[6] Currently the Revised Cardiac Risk Index (RCRI) is used by many cardiologists (**Table 1**).[7]

The importance of familiarity with these types of classifications is not to necessarily be able to classify the patient's cardiac risk, but to know the important questions and parameters on which classification is based. This allows the foot and ankle surgeon a better mechanism to identify patients with underlying cardiac disease and patients

Table 1
Revised cardiac risk index

Revised Cardiac Risk Index	Derivation Set (n = 2893)		Validation Set (n = 1422)	
	Crude Data	Adjusted OR (95% CI)	Crude Data	Adjusted OR (95% CI)
1. High-risk type of surgery	27/894 (3%)	2.8 (1.6, 4.9)	18/490 (4%)	2.6 (1.3, 5.3)
2. Ischemic heart disease	34/951 (4%)	2.4 (1.3, 4.2)	26/478 (5%)	3.8 (1.7, 8.2)
3. History of congestive heart failure	23/434 (5%)	1.9 (1.1,3.5)	19/255 (7%)	4.3 (2.1,8.8)
4. History of cerebrovascular disease	17/291 (6%)	3.2 (1.8, 6.0)	10/140 (7%)	3.0 (1.3, 6.8)
5. Insulin therapy for diabetes	7/112 (6%)	3.0 (1.3, 7.1)	3/59 (5%)	1.0 (0.3, 3.8)
6. Preoperative serum creatinine >2.0 mg/dL	9/103 (9%)	3.0 (1.4, 6.8)	3/55 (5%)	0.9 (0.2, 3.3)

Based on logistic regression models including these 6 variables.
From Lee TH, Marcantonio ER, Mangione CM, et al. Derivation and prospective validation of a simple index for prediction of cardiac risk of major noncardiac surgery. Circulation 1999;100:1047; with permission.

who need cardiology consultation. For example, one of the six clinical factors in the RCRI is "diabetes requiring treatment with insulin prior to surgery." A significant percentage of foot and ankle patients requiring surgery have diabetes and take insulin on a daily basis. The number of predictors from the RCRI and the respective major cardiac complication rates are as follows: 0 predictors, 0.4%; one predictor, 0.9%; two predictors, 6.6%; and three or more predictors, 11%. In this index, a major cardiac complication is defined as MI, pulmonary edema, ventricular fibrillation, primary cardiac arrest, and complete heart block.[7] Having diabetes and requiring insulin represents a predictor from the RCRI and more than doubles a patient's risk (from 0.4% to 0.9%) of having one of these potentially disastrous cardiac complications.

Another method for the assessment of cardiac risk evaluates a patient's functional capacity by determining their ability to perform simple activities of daily living. Hlatky and colleagues[8] validated this form of functional capacity measurement as it correlates with maximum oxygen use with exercise treadmill testing. Determination of functional capacity corresponds to a patient's capacity to perform simple tasks, such as climbing a flight of stairs or walking around the block at a brisk pace. Metabolic equivalencies (METs) or energy expenditures are assigned to such tasks in the following fashion: low-level activities, such as eating, walking, and dressing, range from 1 to 4 METs; moderate level, such as brisk walking, climbing stairs, or playing golf, are given 4 to 10 METs; and strenuous activity, such as tennis or swimming, exceed 10 METs (**Fig. 1**).

Reilly and colleagues[9] followed 600 patients after 612 major surgeries and demonstrated that patients who were unable to climb two flights of stairs or walk four blocks were considered to have exercise intolerance and were more apt to develop cardiovascular complications. In this study exercise intolerance predicted serious complications independent of other patient factors, such as age and tobacco history. Complications were inversely proportional to the number of blocks a patient could walk or the number of flights of stairs a patient could climb. An increase in cardiac risk is present when a patient cannot meet oxygen demands for the performance of activity equivalent to four METs.[5] This becomes an easy task of preoperatively evaluating a patient's functional capacity by having the patient fill out a questionnaire or

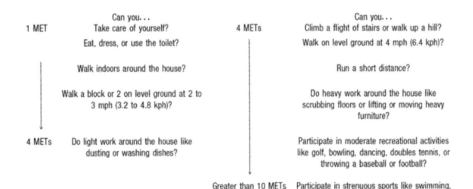

Fig. 1. Duke Activity Status Index. (*Adapted from* Hlatky MA, Boineau RE, Higginbotham MB, et al. A brief self-administered questionnaire to determine functional capacity (the Duke Activity Status Index). Am J Cardiol 1989;64:651–4; with permission.)

asking questions related to the previously mentioned METs and a patient's ability to perform correlative tasks. This process is extremely useful in younger age group patients (30–50) without significant documented medical history where there is low suspicion of potential cardiac history and age may not mandate a preoperative electrocardiogram (ECG). This simple tool can serve as an effective screening procedure to identify cardiac risk in the previously stated patient demographic without which identification may not be ascertained (**Fig. 2**).

The American College of Cardiology/American Heart Association (ACC/AHA) perioperative guidelines were revised and recently published in 2014.[10] These guidelines are structured on evidence-based medicine and give a clear pathway on how to stratify risk and manage patients undergoing noncardiac surgeries in a seven-step approach.

1. Common risk factors for coronary artery disease (CAD), such as personal history of peripheral artery disease, family history of CAD, firsthand or secondhand exposure to tobacco products, hypertension, obesity, hyperlipidemia, and physical inactivity, should be elicited in every patient. In hospitalized patients scheduled for surgery with risk factors for or known CAD, the urgency of surgery predicates the timing of surgery. In patients with open fractures, nonreducible closed, fracture dislocations, and sepsis-related foot infections, surgery is emergent in nature. In these instances, surgery should proceed; however, there should be an evaluation of clinical risk factors that may influence perioperative management and appropriate monitoring and management strategies should be implemented to minimize any perioperative risk of cardiac events. One of the advantages of taking care of pathology affecting the distal lower extremity is this lends itself to different anesthesia approaches, which allows for the safe and comfortable completion of surgery, but do not carry the same attendant, cardiac risks associated with general or even neuraxial anesthesia. With an emergent situation in a patient with a significant history for cardiac disease, it is essential to consult anesthesia and cardiology. In these instances, anesthesia can be provided via a true regional approach, such as a popliteal and saphenous nerve block. This provides adequate anesthesia for the completion of most foot and ankle procedures and a sterile calf tourniquet is used to provide a bloodless field if so desired. If the type of procedure does not lend itself to a calf tourniquet, such as an open pilon fracture with application of

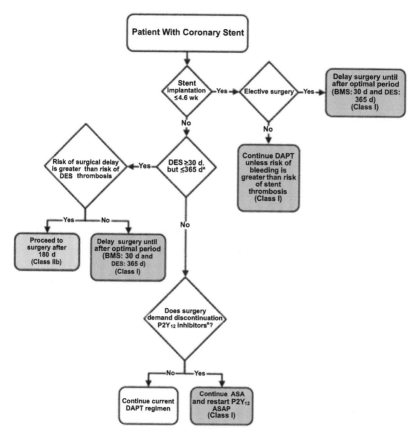

Fig. 2. Proposed algorithm for antiplatelet management in patients with PCI and noncardiac surgery.[a] Assuming patient is currently on DAPT. ASA, aspirin; ASAP, as soon as possible; BMS, bare-metal stent; DAPT, dual antiplatelet therapy; DES, drug-eluting stent; PCI, percutaneous coronary intervention. (*From* Fleisher LA, Fleischmann KE, Auerbach AD, et al. 2014 ACC/AHA guideline on perioperative cardiovascular evaluation and management of patients undergoing noncardiac surgery: a report of the American College of Cardiology/American Heart Association Task Force on practice guidelines. J Am Col Cardiol 2014;64(22):e77–137; with permission.)

external fixator, then a more proximal peripheral nerve block is required. Cardiology consultation is still prudent in these situations because many of these patients need to be non–weight bearing on the affected extremity for a period of time to allow for musculoskeletal healing during postoperative convalescence. Although this may seem insignificant, using a walker or crutches for the performance of activities of daily living, such as using the restroom, is medically taxing for many patients and may represent a situation where undue cardiac stress is experienced on a regular basis. It is important to have a cardiac evaluation in these situations to optimize cardiac treatment and assist in avoiding postoperative cardiac events.

2. In surgeries that are urgent or elective, acute coronary syndrome (ACS) needs to be ruled out. ACS includes unstable angina or MI and patients' symptoms include active chest pain or discomfort, shortness of breath, lightheadedness, and diaphoresis. If there is evidence of or concern for ACS cardiology evaluation should be sought. ACS is confirmed by thorough history and physical examination, obtaining

cardiac biomarkers for ischemia, such as checking troponin levels and by obtaining a 12-lead ECG.

3. If the patient has risk factors for stable CAD (ie, established CAD with no ongoing symptoms), then estimate the perioperative risk of MACE (nonfatal stroke, nonfatal MI, and cardiovascular death) based on the combined clinical/and surgical risk. Estimation of this risk is ascertained by using the American College of Surgeons National Surgical Quality Improvement Program risk calculator (http://www.surgicalriskcalculator.com) or incorporating the RCRI for preoperative risk with an estimation of surgical risk (see **Table 1**).

4. If the patient has a low risk of MACE (<1%), then no further testing is needed, and the patient may proceed to surgery.

5. If the patient is at elevated risk of MACE, then determine functional capacity with an objective measure or scale, such as the Duke Activity Status Index. If the patient has moderate, good, or excellent functional capacity ($\geq$4 METs, then proceed to surgery without further evaluation.

6. If the patient has poor (<4 METs) or unknown functional capacity, then the clinician should consult with the patient and perioperative team to determine whether further testing will impact patient decision making (eg, decision to perform original surgery or willingness to undergo coronary artery bypass graft [CABG] or percutaneous coronary intervention [PCI], depending on the results of the test) or perioperative care. If yes, then pharmacologic stress testing is appropriate. In those patients with unknown functional capacity, exercise stress testing may be reasonable to perform. If the stress test is abnormal, consider coronary angiography and revascularization depending on the extent of the abnormal test. The patient can then proceed to surgery with guideline-directed medical therapy (GDMT) or consider alternative strategies, such as noninvasive treatment of the indication for surgery or palliation. If the test is normal, proceed to surgery according to GDMT.

7. If testing will not impact decision making or care, then proceed to surgery according to GDMT or consider alternative strategies, such as noninvasive treatment of the indication for surgery or palliation.

SUPPLEMENTAL PREOPERATIVE EVALUATION

As per ACC guidelines, although obtaining a 12-lead ECG is reasonable for patients with cardiovascular disease, routine use of resting 12-lead ECG is not recommended in asymptomatic patients undergoing low-risk surgery. Obtaining an echocardiogram to assess left ventricle function as part of preoperative work-up is not indicated; however, it is reasonable to obtain one if patient has shortness of breath that cannot be explained otherwise. Routine screening with noninvasive stress testing is not useful for patients at low risk for noncardiac surgery. For patients with elevated risk (as calculated by RCRI) or an unknown functional capacity, it may be reasonable to perform exercise testing to assess functional capacity. If functional capacity is known, however, and is good (>4–10 METs), no further testing is required. If patient is unable to exercise and has unknown or poor functional capacity, it is reasonable to perform pharmacologic stress testing (dobutamine stress echocardiogram or pharmacologic stress with myocardial perfusion imaging). Routine use of preoperative coronary angiography is not recommended.

PERIOPERATIVE THERAPY

There are no prospective randomized controlled trials supporting coronary revascularization, either CABG or PCI, before noncardiac surgery to decrease intraoperative and postoperative cardiac events. In the largest randomized controlled trial, CARP

(Coronary Artery Revascularization Prophylaxis), there were no differences in perioperative and long-term cardiac outcomes with or without preoperative coronary revascularization by CABG or PCI in patients with documented CAD, with the exclusion of those with left main disease, a left ventricular ejection fraction less than 20%, and severe aortic stenosis.[11] PCI should not be performed as a prerequisite in patients who need noncardiac surgery unless it is clearly indicated for high-risk coronary anatomy (eg, left main disease), unstable angina, MI, or life-threatening arrhythmias caused by active ischemia amenable to PCI. If PCI is necessary, then the urgency of the noncardiac surgery and the risk of bleeding and ischemic events, including stent thrombosis, associated with the surgery in a patient taking dual antiplatelet therapy (DAPT) need to be considered. It is not recommended that routine coronary revascularization be performed before noncardiac surgery exclusively to reduce perioperative cardiac events. The cumulative mortality and morbidity risks of the coronary revascularization procedure and the noncardiac surgery should be weighed carefully in light of the individual patient's overall health, functional status, and prognosis.

TIMING OF ELECTIVE NONCARDIAC SURGERY IN PATIENTS WITH PREVIOUS PERCUTANEOUS CORONARY INTERVENTION

In patients who are on aspirin and a platelet P2Y12 receptor blocker after PCI, the premature cessation of one or both drugs is associated with an increased risk of in-stent thrombosis, MI, or death. Elective noncardiac surgery should be delayed 14 days after balloon angioplasty and 30 days after bare-metal stent (BMS) implantation.[12] Whereas, in patients with drug-eluting stent (DES) it should optimally be delayed for 6 months as per ACC/AHA 2016 guidelines on duration of DAPT in patients with CAD.[13] Minor surgical procedures usually do not require cessation of antiplatelet therapy. For minor surgeries bleeding risk should be assessed before stopping antiplatelet therapy. In patients for whom the risk of bleeding is likely to exceed the risk of a perioperative event because of the premature cessation of DAPT, attempt should be made to continue aspirin alone based on POISE 2 trial.[14]

PERIOPERATIVE MEDICAL THERAPY
β-Blockers

If well tolerated, continuation of β-blockers in those who are currently receiving them for longitudinal reasons, particularly when treatment is provided according to GDMT, such as MI or heart failure, is recommended.[15] In patients with intermediate- or high-risk myocardial ischemia noted in preoperative risk stratification tests, or patients with three or more RCRI risk factors (eg, diabetes mellitus, heart failure, CAD, renal insufficiency, cerebral vascular accident), it may be reasonable to begin perioperative β-blockers.[16] β-Blockers, however, should not be initiated on the day of the surgery in β-blocker-naive patients.[17]

Statins

Statins should be continued in patients currently taking statins and scheduled for noncardiac surgery.[18]

α₂-Agonists

Several studies examined the role of α-agonists (clonidine and mivazerol) for perioperative cardiac protection.[19,20] The ACC guidelines do not recommend use of α_2-agonists for prevention of cardiac events in patients who are undergoing noncardiac surgery.

Antiplatelet Agents

The risk of stent thrombosis in the perioperative period for BMS and DES is highest in the first 4 to 6 weeks after stent implantation. Discontinuation of DAPT, particularly in this early period, is a strong risk factor for stent thrombosis. Should urgent or emergency noncardiac surgery be required, a decision to continue aspirin or DAPT should be individualized, with the risk against the benefits of continuing therapy. The risk of stent thrombosis decreases with time and may be at a stable level by 6 months after DES implantation.[21]

ACC recommends the following: in patients undergoing urgent noncardiac surgery during the first 4 to 6 weeks after BMS or DES implantation, DAPT should be continued unless the relative risk of bleeding outweighs the benefit of the prevention of stent thrombosis. In patients who have received coronary stents and must undergo surgical procedures that mandate the discontinuation of P2Y12 platelet receptor–inhibitor therapy, it is recommended that aspirin be continued if possible and the P2Y12 platelet receptor–inhibitor be restarted as soon as possible after surgery. Management of the perioperative antiplatelet therapy should be determined by a consensus of the surgeon, anesthesiologist, cardiologist, and patient, who should weigh the relative risk of bleeding versus prevention of stent thrombosis. In patients undergoing nonemergency/nonurgent noncardiac surgery who have not had previous coronary stenting, it may be reasonable to continue aspirin when the risk of potential increased cardiac events outweighs the risk of increased bleeding. Initiation or continuation of aspirin is not beneficial in patients undergoing elective noncardiac noncarotid surgery who have not had previous coronary stenting, unless the risk of ischemic events outweighs the risk of surgical bleeding.

Anticoagulants

The risks of bleeding for any surgical procedure must be weighed against the benefit of remaining on anticoagulants on a case-by-case basis. In some instances, in which there is minimal to no risk of bleeding, such as cataract surgery or minor dermatologic procedures, it may be reasonable to continue anticoagulation perioperatively. Patients with prosthetic valves taking vitamin K antagonists may require bridging therapy with either unfractionated heparin or low-molecular-weight heparin, depending on the location of the prosthetic valve and associated risk factors for thrombotic and thromboembolic events. For patients with a mechanical mitral valve, regardless of the absence of additional risk factors for thromboembolism, or patients with an aortic valve and one or more additional risk factor (eg, atrial fibrillation, previous thromboembolism, left ventricular dysfunction, hypercoagulable condition, or an older-generation prosthetic aortic valve), bridging anticoagulation may be appropriate when interruption of anticoagulation for perioperative procedures is required and control of hemostasis is essential.[22] For patients with atrial fibrillation and normal renal function undergoing elective procedures during which hemostatic control is essential, such as major surgery, spine surgery, and epidural catheterization, discontinuation of anticoagulants for greater than or equal to 48 hours is suggested. There have been no studies on the benefit of anticoagulants on the prevention of perioperative myocardial ischemia or MI.

PERIOPERATIVE MANAGEMENT OF PATIENTS WITH CARDIOVASCULAR IMPLANTABLE ELECTRONIC DEVICES

To assist clinicians with the perioperative evaluation and management of patients with pacemakers and implantable cardioverter-defibrillators (ICDs), the Heart Rhythm

Society and the American Society of Anesthesiologists together developed an expert consensus statement that was published in July 2011 and endorsed by the ACC and the AHA.[23]

The major issue in patients with permanent pacemakers or ICDs is the potential for electromagnetic interference. The intensity of electromagnetic interference from cauterization is related to the direction and distance of the current to the pacemaker generator and leads. If the cautery is to be used near the generator, care should be taken to avoid loss of ventricular pacing, causing asystole. If possible, the surgeon should use bipolar cautery, which, unlike unipolar cautery, disperses energy over a small surface area.[24] The surgeon should use the lowest possible amplitude and apply the current in bursts rather than continuously. If the patient has an ICD, the device may interpret electrocautery as ventricular fibrillation, leading to an unnecessary shock. To avoid such problems, defibrillatory function should be turned off immediately before surgery, and turned on just afterward, whereas pacing function should remain on. An external defibrillator should be immediately available and switched on, with defibrillation patches in place on the patient.[25]

SUMMARY

For the foot and ankle surgeon, the most important step in dealing with a patient with cardiac disease is performing a complete history and physical with careful attention directed toward the identification of risks factors associated with cardiac disease, specifically CAD. Risk stratification plays a primary role in appropriate placement of a specific patient toward predilection of developing perioperative cardiac problems. The entire process also identifies factors that can be improved on or even eliminated, thus decreasing the likelihood of cardiac events associated with surgery. This cardiac optimization is a by-product of coordinated care and appropriate cardiology involvement.

REFERENCES

1. Weiser TG, Regenbogen SE, Thompson KD, et al. An estimation of the global volume of surgery: a modelling strategy based on available data. Lancet 2008; 372(9633):139–44.
2. Botto F, Alonso-Coello P, Chan MT, et al, Vascular events In noncardiac Surgery patients cOhort evaluatioN (VISION) Writing Group, on behalf of The Vascular events In noncardiac Surgery patients cOhort evaluatioN (VISION) Investigators, Appendix 1. The Vascular events In noncardiac Surgery patients cOhort evaluatioN (VISION) Study Investigators Writing Group, Appendix 2. The Vascular events In noncardiac Surgery patients cOhort evaluatioN Operations Committee, Vascular events In noncardiac Surgery patients cOhort evaluatioN VISION Study. Myocardial injury after noncardiac surgery: a large, international, prospective cohort study establishing diagnostic criteria, characteristics, predictors, and 30-day outcomes. Anesthesiology 2014;120(3):564–78.
3. van Waes JA, Nathoe HM, de Graaff JC, et al. Myocardial injury after noncardiac surgery and its association with short-term mortality. Circulation 2013;127(23): 2264–71.
4. Udeh BL, Dalton JE, Hata JS, et al. Economic trends from 2003 to 2010 for perioperative myocardial infarction: a retrospective, cohort study. Anesthesiology 2014;121(1):36–45.
5. Engberding N, Weitz H. [Chapter 9] Cardiovascular disease. In: Lubin MF, Dodson TF, Winawer NH, editors. Medical management of the surgical patient.

A textbook of perioperative medicine. 5th edition. New York: Cambridge University Press; 2013. p. 75–92.

6. Goldman L, Caldera DL, Nussbaum SR, et al. Multifactorial index of cardiac risk in noncardiac surgical procedures. N Engl J Med 1977;297:845–50.

7. Lee TH, Marcantonio ER, Mangione CM, et al. Derivation and prospective validation of a simple index for prediction of cardiac risk of major noncardiac surgery. Circulation 1999;100:1043–9.

8. Hlatky MA, Boineau RE, Higginbotham MB, et al. A brief self-administered questionnaire to determine functional capacity (the Duke Activity Status Index). Am J Cardiol 1989;64:651–4.

9. Reilly DF, McNeely MJ, Doerner D, et al. Self-reported exercise tolerance and the risk of serious perioperative complications. Arch Intern Med 1999;159:2185–92.

10. Fleisher LA, Fleischmann KE, Auerbach AD, et al. 2014 ACC/AHA guideline on perioperative cardiovascular evaluation and management of patients undergoing noncardiac surgery: a report of the American College of Cardiology/American Heart Association Task Force on Practice Guidelines. J Am Coll Cardiol 2014; 64(22):e77–137.

11. McFalls EO, Ward HB, Moritz TE, et al. Coronary-artery revascularization before elective major vascular surgery. N Engl J Med 2004;351(27):2795–804.

12. Kałuza GL, Joseph J, Lee JR, et al. Catastrophic outcomes of noncardiac surgery soon after coronary stenting. J Am Coll Cardiol 2000;35(5):1288–94.

13. Levine GN, Bates ER, Bittl JA, et al. 2016 ACC/AHA guideline focused update on duration of dual antiplatelet therapy in patients with coronary artery disease: a report of the American College of Cardiology/American Heart Association Task Force on Clinical Practice Guidelines. J Am Coll Cardiol 2016;68(10):1082–115.

14. Devereaux PJ, Mrkobrada M, Sessler DI, et al. Aspirin in patients undergoing noncardiac surgery. N Engl J Med 2014;370(16):1494–503.

15. London MJ, Hur K, Schwartz GG, et al. Association of perioperative beta-blockade with mortality and cardiovascular morbidity following major noncardiac surgery. JAMA 2013;309:1704–13.

16. Boersma E, Poldermans D, Bax JJ, et al. Predictors of cardiac events after major vascular surgery: role of clinical characteristics, dobutamine echocardiography, and beta-blocker therapy. JAMA 2001;285:1865–73.

17. POISE Trial Investigators. Rationale, design, and organization of the PeriOperative ISchemic Evaluation (POISE) trial: a randomized controlled trial of metoprolol versus placebo in patients undergoing noncardiac surgery. Am Heart J 2006; 152(2):223–30.

18. Durazzo AES, Machado FS, Ikeoka DT, et al. Reduction in cardiovascular events after vascular surgery with atorvastatin: a randomized trial. J Vasc Surg 2004;39: 967–75.

19. Oliver MF, Goldman L, Julian DG, et al. Effect of mivazerol on perioperative cardiac complications during non-cardiac surgery in patients with coronary heart disease the European Mivazerol Trial (EMIT). Anesthesiology 1999;91(4):951.

20. Stühmeier KD, Mainzer B, Cierpka J, et al. Small, oral dose of clonidine reduces the incidence of intraoperative myocardial ischemia in patients having vascular surgery. Anesthesiology 1996;85:706–12.

21. Tokushige A, Shiomi H, Morimoto T, et al. Incidence and outcome of surgical procedures after coronary bare-metal and drug-eluting stent implantation: a report from the CREDO-Kyoto PCI/CABG registry cohort-2. Circ Cardiovasc Interv 2012;5(2):237–46.

22. Nishimura RA, Otto CM, Bonow RO, et al. 2014 AHA/ACC guideline for the management of patients with valvular heart disease: a report of the American College of Cardiology/American Heart Association Task Force on Practice Guidelines. Circulation 2014;129:e521–643.
23. Crossley GH, Poole JE, Rozner MA, et al. The Heart Rhythm Society (HRS)/American Society of Anesthesiologists (ASA) expert consensus statement on the perioperative management of patients with implantable defibrillators, pacemakers and arrhythmia monitors: facilities and patient management. Developed as a joint project with the American Society of Anesthesiologists (ASA), and in collaboration with the American Heart Association (AHA), and the Society of Thoracic Surgeons (STS). Heart Rhythm 2011;8:1114–54.
24. Cheng A, Nazarian S, Spragg DD, et al. Effects of surgical and endoscopic electrocautery on modern-day permanent pacemaker and implantable cardioverter-defibrillator systems. Pacing Clin Electrophysiol 2008;31(3):344–50.
25. Hauser RG, Kallinen L. Deaths associated with implantable cardioverter defibrillator failure and deactivation reported in the United States Food and Drug Administration manufacturer and user facility device experience database. Heart Rhythm 2004;1:399–405.

Perioperative Management of the Rheumatoid Patient

Jesse Wolfe, DPM, Joshua Wolfe, DPM, MHA, H. John Visser, DPM*

KEYWORDS

- Rheumatoid arthritis • Perioperative management • Methotrexate • DMARDs

KEY POINTS

- Perioperative evaluation of rheumatoid patients should be performed from a multidisciplinary approach.
- History and physical examination of rheumatoid patients should focus on their current disease state, comorbidities, and pharmacologic therapy.
- Rheumatoid medications should be assessed in the perioperative setting according to recent guidelines.
- Patient education on potential complications and postoperative expectations is necessary.

INTRODUCTION

Rheumatoid arthritis (RA) is an inflammatory arthritis more prevalent in women than men and affects 0.5% to 1.0% of the population.[1,2] Hallmark disease characteristics of RA include chronic symmetric destructive polyarticular synovitis of the hands and feet. Other extra-articular manifestations also may be present involving both small and large joints, with exception for the distal phalangeal joints of the hand and noncervical spine. These RA-targeted joints lead to deformities, including ulnar deviation, as well as boutonniere and swan-neck deformities in the hands. Foot involvement affects the forefoot primarily and proceeds in most cases to the hindfoot and ankle. Targeted joints include the proximal interphalangeal joints (PIPJ) and metatarsophalangeal joints (MPJ) in the forefoot, whereas the subtalar joint (STJ) and talonavicular joint (TNJ) are commonly affected in the hindfoot.[1] Due to the RA disease process, various surgical procedures are often performed, such as joint arthroplasty, tendon reconstruction, rheumatoid nodule removal, tarsal tunnel and carpal tunnel decompression, and intrathoracic nodule biopsy.[1] Fortunately, pharmacologic therapy, such as

Disclosure Statements: Drs J. Wolfe and J. Wolfe have no disclosures. Dr H.J. Visser has no conflicts to disclose pertaining to this paper.
Foot and Ankle Surgery Residency, SSM Health DePaul Hospital, 12303 DePaul Drive, Suite B1, St Louis, MO 63044, USA
* Corresponding author. 11709 Old Ballas Road, Suite 202, St Louis, MO 63141.
E-mail address: tsarhjv@aol.com

disease-modifying antirheumatic drugs (DMARDs), nonsteroidal anti-inflammatory drugs (NSAIDs), analgesics, and corticosteroids, have reduced disease progression and severity of RA-associated conditions over the years. DMARDs have also revolutionized the standards of care for patients with RA. Early diagnosis and effective treatment have been shown to induce rapid recession.[3] Nevertheless, a thorough preoperative evaluation of patients with RA is necessary regardless of disease remission or pharmacologic control of clinical symptoms.

Perioperative management of patients with RA should be performed from a multidisciplinary approach due to the complexity of the rheumatic disease process. This multidisciplinary team should include rheumatologists, anesthesiologists, cardiologists, and hematologists, due to potential RA-associated comorbidities.[2] A few examples of these comorbidities include fatigue, anemia, Felty syndrome, interstitial lung disease, pleural effusions, neuropathies, vasculopathies, coronary artery disease, pericarditis, adenopathy, scleritis, Sjögren syndrome, cervical spine disease, and cricoarytenoid arthritis.[4] Multiple RA treatment guidelines have been proposed for medical and perioperative management of patients undergoing elective surgery in an effort to reduce complications.[5–9] These proposed guidelines aid the surgeon in minimizing the risk of iatrogenic and postoperative complications.

PREOPERATIVE CONSIDERATIONS
History and Physical

A comprehensive history and physical should be performed preoperatively. Pertinent details within the patient's history include age, disease duration, functional status, specific joint involvement, and extra-articular manifestations. The history also should include a complete medication list that addresses medication duration, steroid use, prior surgical complications, and other associated comorbidities.[4] In addition to the normal preoperative examination, an emphasis on posture, gait, joint mobility, and integument integrity should be considered in the patient with RA.

Preoperative Testing

Appropriate routine preoperative testing may be useful in gaining an understanding of the disease progression among patients with RA, particularly in those who have a prolonged history of DMARD, NSAID, and corticosteroid use.

A complete blood count should be considered when risk of significant blood loss is present. Patients with RA often may present with comorbidities such as mild hypochromatic anemia and medication side effects, including drug-related anemia, leukopenia, and bone marrow suppression.[4] These patients should have their hemoglobin monitored preoperatively and postoperatively, as a transfusion may be necessary pending the amount of blood loss during the procedure.

A complete metabolic profile also should be considered in the presence of hepatorenal impairment secondary to antirheumatic medications. Other routine preoperative testing may include urinalysis, urine culture, 12-lead electrocardiogram in patients older than 40, and chest radiographs in patients older than 50. Preoperative assessment of other medical comorbidities is prudent in reducing surgical morbidity and mortality complications.[4,10–13]

Comorbidities

Recognition of the systemic effects of RA is imperative to an appropriate preoperative evaluation. Specifically, assessment and screening for RA-associated cervical, cardiac, and pulmonary diseases may serve to decrease the likelihood of adverse postoperative complications.

CERVICAL ASSESSMENT
Atlantoaxial Instability

Cervical spine involvement of patients with RA ranges between 25% and 86% and poses a risk for spinal cord injury during intubation for airway management.[14,15] Documentation of cervical spine disease with or without neurologic involvement is necessary. This is because 80% of patients with RA presenting with radiographic evidence of cervical spine disease; however, 50% are asymptomatic[16,17] and 36% of symptomatic patients demonstrate concurrent neurologic progression.[18] It is important for either a neurologist or the anesthesiologist to perform a complete neurologic examination in these patients preoperatively to understand the clinical level of neurologic manifestations of the cervical spine RA involvement and, just as importantly, to establish a neurologic baseline to which any postoperative changes can be compared.

Three common RA cervical spine deformities are observed, with atlantoaxial subluxation being the most common (65%) followed by superior migration of the odontoid (20%) and subaxial subluxation (15%).[14,15] Atlantoaxial subluxation may be present in the hypermobile neck of a rheumatoid patient and a preoperative evaluation is necessary. Higher incidence of atlantoaxial subluxation has been noted particularly in individuals with long-standing history of the disease with peripheral joint erosion, prolonged corticosteroid therapy, cervical symptoms, and subcutaneous nodules.[4] Superior migration of the odontoid, also known as atlantoaxial impaction, is secondary to erosion of the occiput and C1-C2 joints. This results in direct compression of the brainstem by the odontoid process and may result in neurologic injury or death. Subaxial subluxation is a "stepladder" deformity usually associated with kyphosis. This occurs at multiple levels of the neck, especially if the patient has a history of previous cervical fusions.[14,16]

Standard static cervical radiographic views as well as dynamic lateral radiographs demonstrating flexion and extension should be obtained preoperatively in patients with inflammatory arthropathies to assess for C1-C2 instability. Radiographs also should be obtained in patients with a history of neck pain with or without crepitus on range of motion, such as a positive L'Hermitte sign, and in cases of radicular nerve pain and limb weakness.[14,19]

The anterior atlantodental interval (AADI) is the most common measurement to evaluate for this deformity. Normal values are less than 3 mm between the atlas (C1) and odontoid process (C2). If instability is present, this measurement will increase on the lateral flexion view. Although the AADI is nonspecific to determining presence of neurologic deficits, it is helpful in determining if further workup for atlantoaxial instability is necessary in the perioperative rheumatoid patient.[14]

In cases in which the AADI is greater than 2.5 mm, the anesthesiologist must be notified preoperatively. In patients with a known history of atlantoaxial instability, it is important to recognize the development of any new neurologic symptoms. The atlantoaxial instability is a progressive deformity that, if left untreated, can progress until the ring of the atlas is disrupted. This results in compression of the posterior spinal cord, further predisposing the perioperative patient to neurologic injury. When neurologic symptoms are present, MRI should be obtained to evaluate for further spinal cord compression.[14] Additional precautions may be necessary in the perioperative patient, including a soft cervical collar and minimal manipulation during transport. Although, it should be noted that the soft cervical collar does not function as a protective device, rather as a reminder of the cervical instability present.[14]

Cricoarytenoid Arthritis

Cricoarytenoid arthritis (CA) is a well-known condition present in 26% to 86% of the RA population.[20] Despite the high prevalence of CA, acute airway compromise remains a rare but life-threatening complication within this population. The cricoarytenoid joint is the articulation between cricoid cartilages at the lateral aspect of the posterior lamina and the arytenoid. This joint functions as a ball and socket and is responsible for facilitating respiration, airway protection, and phonation.[20] Patients with RA who present with throat tension, fullness, hoarseness, odynophagia, or pain with speaking should be evaluated for CA, preoperatively. Pain radiating to the ears due to impingement of the glossopharyngeal and vagus nerves by the CA joint also may be present. If chronic, CA may be asymptomatic or even misdiagnosed as chronic bronchitis or asthma. In the perioperative patient with RA, CA can result in acute airway compromise during the intubation or extubation period, requiring a tracheostomy as a life-saving measure.[20]

Cardiovascular Assessment

Understanding the factors associated with cardiovascular disease (CVD) and how it relates to the rheumatoid patient is imperative for the podiatric surgeon to understand before surgical intervention. Individuals with RA, as well as other inflammatory joint disorders, are at a significantly elevated risk for mortality related to CVD. These individuals have approximately a 50% increase in CVD mortality in comparison with the general population.[21] Therefore, this elevated mortality rate lends to the need for appropriate risk management of the rheumatoid patient. In addition, the individual with RA who does not have clinical evidence for CVD has still been shown to have an increased in cardiac complications, such as left ventricular diastolic dysfunction, in comparison with the general population.[22]

Although the correlation is not clear-cut, the more severe the inflammation associated with RA disease activity, the greater the impact on cardiovascular risk.[2] Several studies have demonstrated links between RA and CVD. A meta-analysis, illustrated a relative risk increase in overall CVD, all-cause early mortality, and cardiovascular mortality when compared with nonrheumatoid patients.[23] Another study reported similar cardiovascular findings that patients with RA experience elevated myocardial infarctions (both unrecognized and hospitalized) and have a greater history of angina compared with nonrheumatoid patients.[24] Surprisingly, patients with RA with low disease activity and no history suggestive of CVD have cardiovascular-associated death.[25] It is apparent that patients with RA have an increased mortality risk associated with CVD, stressing the importance of early recognition, treatment, and optimization of these patients.

Cardiovascular risk management in the patient with RA must take into account a variety of factors. First, an electrocardiogram is an important diagnostic tool that should be used preoperatively in the patient with RA to evaluate overt arrhythmias, but also to evaluate QTc intervals. Patients with RA are specifically at risk for QTc prolongation, which is a prognostic sign for arrythmias and sudden cardiac death.[25] In addition a 50-m increase in the QTc interval has been related to increasing the risk of all-cause mortality to twice that of the general population.[25] Second, although the use of the Systemic Coronary Risk Evaluation (SCORE) to predict a CVD event within 10 years is not necessarily within the purview of the podiatric surgeon, it is a useful prognostic tool that may benefit the surgeon.[26] The use of the SCORE for CVD must also be multiplied by a factor of 1.5 to account for the 50% increase in risk associated with RA in comparison with the general population.[21,26] Third, the evaluation of the inflammatory process within the patient with RA is an excellent marker for disease progression. A major cardiovascular dysfunction associated with RA and elevated inflammatory markers is carotid intima media thickness. Although the clinical utility of this measurement is less applicable, it is important to be aware of this connection as an additional risk factor for the patient with RA.[26]

RA is a multifactorial disease that affects many areas, including the cardiovascular arena. Although the podiatric surgeon does not necessarily manage these cardiovascular complications, it is important to recognize this RA-associated comorbidity. A holistic understanding of the rheumatoid patient allows for more effective integration of the podiatric surgeon in the multidisciplinary team.

Pulmonary Assessment

Over the past several decades, research on the RA disease process has focused on joint inflammation and extra-articular manifestations. Interestingly, multiple pulmonary diseases also have been found to be associated with RA, including interstitial lung disease and drug-induced lung disease secondary to prolonged DMARD use.

One theory on the development of pulmonary disease in patients with RA is due to the development of anti-cyclic citrullinated peptide (CCP) antibodies. CCPs develop from a posttranslational modification of peptidyl arginine deaminase-1 and peptidyl arginine deaminase-2, converting arginine to citrulline.[27] This results in increasing immunogenicity of the protein and has been associated with other inflammatory disease states, such as psoriasis, idiopathic pulmonary fibrosis, and multiple sclerosis.[27] Likewise vimentin, filaggrin, and fibronectin synovial proteins can become citrullinated, and as result antibodies develop and are thought to be associated with the development of RA-associated pulmonary diseases.[27] This is due to the significant association between CCPs found in joint inflammation and multiple RA airway diseases, such as bronchial wall thickening and pulmonary nodules.[27,28]

Rheumatoid Arthritis Interstitial Lung Disease

The most common cause of RA pulmonary-related mortality and morbidity is RA interstitial lung disease (RA-ILD). Often, RA-ILD has a presentation suggestive of idiopathic interstitial pneumonia and is difficult to differentiate. Acute respiratory symptoms of the patient with RA in the perioperative setting should not be taken lightly and further workup is warranted.[27]

Drug-Induced Lung Disease

DMARDs have become a mainstay therapy in the treatment of RA; however, they pose their own risk in the form of drug-induced lung disease. Infection, airway disease, and nodules are known associations of DMARDs.[27,28] Other serious side effects specific to biological DMARDs include pulmonary toxicity, which when present, has a mortality rate of 35.5%.[27,29–32]

Medication Considerations

Individuals with RA often use a wide variety of medications that have the potential to affect the patient intraoperatively as well as in the postoperative period. It is important to understand the effects and implications that these medications can have on the patient with RA during the surgical period.[33] The most common medications prescribed in patients with RA are NSAIDs, steroids, DMARDs, and biological agents. Many of these medications are used in combination therapy.[33] The prevalence of patients with RA undergoing arthroplasty while on a traditional or biologic DMARD medication is estimated to be between 75% and 84%. Similarly, corticosteroid use is estimated to be 80% within the same population.[34,35]

One of the most debated topics related to patients with RA revolves around the perioperative protocol for the variety of drugs used to treat this inflammatory disease process. These medications can be very complicated. Also, recommendations regarding starting and stopping medications around a surgery is ever changing. As an example, in the past, methotrexate was discontinued 2 weeks before surgery and then resumed 2 weeks after surgery to avoid infection. In general, this is no longer recommended; however, this remains a debated topic. It is important to understand that each patient is different and has had an individual response to their particular anti-RA regimen. It is essential that the rheumatologist, surgeon, and, perhaps, infectious disease specialist collaborate on the perioperative management of each patient's anti-RA drug therapy. It can be extremely debilitating to a patient with RA to have the medication regimen altered perioperatively, and this should be minimized if at all possible and consideration should be given to acceptable alternative medications to replace discontinued perioperative medications. This will potentially lessen the effect of discontinuing a needed medication and allow for continued mobility in the perioperative period.

Nonsteroidal Anti-inflammatory Drugs and Acetylsalicylic Acid Recommendations

NSAID use in management of RA symptoms is a traditional treatment modality. Due to the nonselective inhibitory effect on Thromboxane A2 in platelet aggregation, an increased surgical bleeding risk is present and should be discontinued. In the use of NSAIDs, platelet function is reversibly inhibited and return to platelet function is derived on the drug half-life. In anticipation of a surgical procedure, the NSAID should be discontinued 4 to 5 half-lives before surgery to allow a return to proper hemostasis. As a general guideline, discontinuing any NSAIDs 5 days before surgery is adequate, with the exception of piroxicam, due to its prolonged average half-life of 50 hours (range 14–158 hours) and should be discontinued 10 days in advance of a surgical procedure.[1]

Aspirin (acetylsalicylic acid) irreversibly binds to platelet cyclooxygenase and thus does not rely on half-life duration for return of platelet aggregation function. Instead, a return to platelet aggregation is achieved by the body's own platelet production through totipotent stem cells. This results in the formation of megakaryocytes and eventually thrombocytes (platelets) regulated by thrombopoietin produced in the liver and kidneys. Aspirin should be withheld 10 days before surgery to allow for adequate formation of new platelets.[1]

Synthetic Disease-Modifying Antirheumatic Drugs

The treatment methodology for individuals with RA has evolved significantly as the disease progression for RA has become better understood, but controversy remains within some areas of the literature. Synthetic DMARDs are among the most common medications prescribed for the rheumatoid patient and are considered to be the frontline medication, specifically methotrexate, among recent literature.[36] Synthetic DMARDs pertains to methotrexate, sulfasalazine, leflunomide, and hydroxychloroquine.[37]

The mechanism of action (MOA) of the synthetic DMARDs are highly variable, but important from a completeness standpoint. The podiatric surgeon should have an understanding of how the MOA pathways affect the patient perioperatively.

Methotrexate has an MOA of inhibiting dihydrofolate reductase (DHFR) which causes a reduction in tetrahydrofolate, ultimately resulting in inhibition of purine and pyrimidine synthesis. Methotrexate has associated toxicities involving bone marrow suppression, liver toxicity, and stomatitis. In addition, methotrexate must be supplemented with folic acid due to the inhibition of DHFR and the folate pathway.[38] Methotrexate potentiates adenosine production resulting in inhibition of cytokine, lymphocytes, and monocyte production leading to apoptosis.[39,40] In addition, the use of methotrexate has been shown in the literature to not have adverse effects perioperatively and therefore does not need to be discontinued for surgery.[35,40–42] Recent guidelines published by the American College of Rheumatology in conjunction with the American Association of Hip and Knee Surgeons advocate for continuation of methotrexate through the operative period.[5] The primary exception to this recommendation would be for the patient with a delayed union or nonunion. The literature is controversial regarding whether inhibition of osteoblastic activity by methotrexate occurs. Due to this controversy, some literature still recommends discontinuing methotrexate use 1 week preoperatively and 1 to 2 weeks postoperatively.[40,43–45]

Sulfasalazine (SSZ) is an inhibitor for de novo pyrimidine synthesis via selective inhibition of dihydro-orotate dehydrogenase.[46,47] SSZ is a combination of 5-aminosalicylic acid and sulfapyridine via an azo bond. Sulfasalazine was initially used for RA due to its anti-inflammatory and antimicrobial properties and continues to be used in combination therapy.[47–49] The American College of Rheumatology (ACR)/American Association of Hip and Knee Surgeons (AAHK) guidelines recommend continuing SSZ throughout the perioperative period.[5]

Hydroxychloroquine (HCQ) while most commonly known for its use as an antimalarial drug, also is used within DMARD treatments for RA. The MOA for HCQ is still relatively unknown, but studies have shown involvement with 3 areas: inhibition of lysosomal activity, antigen presentation, and Toll-like receptor signaling.[50,51] Studies have exhibited multiple positive attributes for patients with RA from HCQ therapy, such as decreasing lipid profiles, CVD risk, rate of diabetes, HgA1c, and overall rate of cardiovascular events.[51] ACR/AAHK guidelines recommend continuing HCQ through the perioperative period.[5]

Leflunomide is a de novo pyrimidine synthesis inhibitor that is rapidly absorbed after oral administration. Leflunomide is subsequently altered to its active state, malononitrilamide, also known as teriflunomide. Teriflunomide inhibits ribonucleotide uridine monophosphate pyrimidine (rUMP), a specific pyrimidine within the RA pathway. rUMP is specifically inhibited by decreasing dihydro-orotate dehydrogenase, a mitochondrial enzyme.[52–54] The literature has shown that patients on leflunomide have a significantly elevated risk for postoperative infection. Therefore, leflunomide should be discontinued 1 to 2 days before surgery. If needed, cholestyramine may be used to rapidly lower parenteral leflunomide levels to prevent surgical complications. Leflunomide may be restarted within 1 to 2 weeks, postoperatively, once the incision is well-coapted.[40,55,56] These synthetic DMARD medications are summarized in **Table 1**.

Glucocorticoids

Glucocorticoids have been accepted as an adjunctive medication to be used in combination with DMARDs. Due to the fast-acting nature of glucocorticoids, steroids are often used as bridging therapy during the latency period before DMARDs reaching their effective dose.[40] Despite this, recent systematic reviews have examined the literature and demonstrated that there is a lack of specific recommendations for glucocorticoid treatment.[57] In addition, glucocorticoids are not without associated risks. The most concerning potential complications are surgical site infections, impaired wound healing, decreased bone quality, and hemodynamic instability secondary to adrenal insufficiency from hypothalamus-pituitary-adrenal axis suppression.[40,58] One of the greatest concerns to the podiatric surgeon is postoperative infection. One study in

Table 1
Synthetic DMARD medications

Synthetic DMARD	Mechanism of Action	Preoperative Management	Postoperative Management
Methotrexate	Inhibition of dihydrofolate reductase[79]	Discontinue 1 wk before surgery[5]; some literature recommends maintaining usual dosage[79]	Resume 1–2 wk after surgery[5]; some literature recommends maintaining usual dosage[79]
Leflunomide	De novo pyrimidine synthesis inhibitor via selective inhibition of rUMP, using active agent terifluonmide[79]	Discontinue 1–2 d before surgery[5]; some literature recommends discontinuing 2 wk before surgery[79]	Resume 1–2 wk after surgery, once the incision is well-coapted[5]; some literature recommends resuming 3 d after surgery[79]
Sulfasalazine	Inhibits de novo pyrimidine synthesis via selective inhibition of dihydro-orotate dehydrogenase[79]	Maintain usual dosage[5]	Maintain usual dosage[5]
Hydroxychloroquine	Stabilizes lysosomal membranes, reduces IL-1 and TNF synthesis[79]	Maintain usual dosage[79]	Maintain usual dosage[79]
Ciclosporin	Inhibits T-cell activation via calcineurin-cyclophilin ligand inhibition.[79]	Maintain usual dosage[79]	Maintain usual dosage[79]
Mycophenolate mofetil	Inhibits B-cell and T-cell proliferation via purine[79]	Discontinue 2 wk before surgery[79]	Resume 1–2 wk after surgery[79]
Azathioprine	Inhibits purine synthesis[79]	Maintain usual dosage[79]	Maintain usual dosage[79]

Abbreviations: APC, activated Protein C; DMARD, disease-modifying antirheumatic drug; IL, interleukin; rUMP, ribonucleotide uridine monophosphate pyrimidine; TNF, tumor necrosis factor.

Data from Franco AS, Iuamoto LR, Pereira RMR. Perioperative management of drugs commonly used in patients with rheumatic diseases: a review. Clinics (Sao Paulo) 2017;72(6);386–90; and Goodman SM, Springer B, Guyatt G, et al. 2017 American College of Rheumatology/American Association of Hip and Knee Surgeons guideline for the perioperative management of antirheumatic medication in patients with rheumatic diseases undergoing elective total hip or total knee arthroplasty. Arthritis Care Res (Hoboken) 2017;69(8):1111–24; with permission.

the orthopedic literature found that individuals receiving more than 15 mg of steroid daily were at a much higher risk, 20 times that of the general population, for postoperative infection in arthroplasty patients.[58] Due to decreasing bone quality with prolonged steroid therapy, some literature recommends adjunctive therapy using Teriparatide to improve bone mineral density as well as decrease fracture risk.[40,59,60] The literature recommends that individuals undergoing glucocorticoid therapy for RA should be tapered to an appropriate preoperative dose, while also preventing the risk of Addisonian crisis via adrenal insufficiency and also preventing postoperative infection from diminished wound healing.[40,61,62] Although the literature suggests that doses be less than 15 mg per day of steroid, specifically prednisolone in this instance, the literature does have controversy and lacks concrete evidence to support recommendations for particular dosing strategies.[57,58] Therefore, it is important for the surgeon to have an ongoing conversation with rheumatology regarding perioperative management of corticosteroids in the patient with RA. This same discussion should take place with the anesthesiologist to discuss the potential administration of supplemental perioperative steroids to avoid hypotension related to suppressed endogenous adrenal function in patients who have received daily corticosteroid therapy.

Biologic Disease-Modifying Antirheumatic Drugs

Biologic DMARDs (bDMARDs) are approached very differently in comparison with other DMARDs. The degree of variation in MOA for bDMARDs creates a situation in which the surgeon must be aware of variations in preoperative and postoperative protocol. bDMARDs are a large group of medications and include tumor necrosis factor (TNF)α inhibitors (etanercepts, adalimumab, infliximab, golimumab, certolizumab), abatacept, rituximab, tocilizumab, clazakizumab, sarilumab, and sirukumab, as well as Janus kinase (JAK) inhibitors (tofacitinib and baricitinib).[5] Due to this variation in mechanisms, this has created variation in recommendations in the literature. The advancements of bDMARDs has led to significant improvements in the management of RA, and the variability has significantly affected perioperative management of the patient with RA. **Table 1** summarizes the bDMARDs, their mechanisms of action, and their perioperative consideration. With regard to TNFα inhibitors, the ACR recommends discontinuing these medications 1 week before surgery, whereas some of the orthopedic literature suggests 1 week before surgery for etanercept or 4 weeks before surgery for adalimumab and infliximab.[5,40] Moreover, these medications are recommended to be restarted at 1 week postoperatively by the ACR, whereas some orthopedic literature suggests 2 weeks to prevent postoperative infection.[40] The overarching theme with stopping and restarting these medications is the event of a rheumatoid flare, extent/risk of surgery, and infection. If an infection is present, without a flare-up, TNFα inhibitors should be discontinued until 1 week after the last sign of infection has resolved.[40] Moreover, it is important that the surgeon communicates with the rheumatologist so that appropriate timing of surgery is in accordance within the RA medication cycle. These biologic DMARD medications are summarized in **Table 2**.

Perioperative Assessment

Assessing the rheumatoid patient in the perioperative setting is important. Patients with RA may present with foot and ankle deformities, including synovitis and pannus formation. This connective tissue disarrangement predisposes the patient to metatarsophalangeal instability, as well as hammer toe and claw toe deformity.[3,63] In patients with a long-standing history of RA-associated deformities, prudent evaluation of soft tissue integrity is necessary.

Infection and Wound Healing

Most common complications following elective foot and ankle surgery in patients with RA are infection and wound healing. Patients with RA have demonstrated an overall wound healing complication rate of 32% and an infection rate of 12% to 14%.[64–67] To avoid these complications, special attention should be payed to achieving hemostasis during the surgery and a low threshold should exist for the utilization of a drain. These patients tend to be bleeders, and precautions should be taken to prevent and

Table 2
Biologic DMARD medications

Biologic DMARD	Mechanism of Action	Perioperative Management
Adalimumab (anti-TNFα)	Binds TNFα, inhibition of Treg[70]	Discontinue 4 wk before surgery; resume 1 wk after surgery
Infliximab (anti-TNFα)	Binds TNFα via monoclonal antibody[71]	Discontinue 4 wk before surgery; resume 1 wk after surgery
Golimumab (anti-TNFα)	Binds TNFα via monoclonal antibody[72]	Discontinue 28 d before surgery[79]; resume 1 wk after surgery
Certolizumab pegol (anti-TNFα)	Binds TNFα via PEGylated anti-TNFα Fab[73]	Discontinue 28 d before surgery[79]; resume 1 wk after surgery
Etanercept (anti-TNFα)	Binds TNFα via TNFα receptor fusion protein[74]	Discontinue 1 wk before surgery; resume 1 wk after surgery
Abatacept	Fusion protein that binds to CD80 and CD86 receptors on APC, resulting in selective inhibition of CD28 leading to T-cell inhibition and B-cell immunologic response[75]	Discontinue 25 d before surgery[79]
Rituximab	Targets CD20 on the surface of B-cells (pre-B through memory B-cells)[76]	Discontinue 100 d before surgery[79]; discontinue 1 mo before surgery[5]
Tocilizumab	Inhibits RA cytokine pathogenesis via an IL-6 receptor antibody[77]	Discontinue 26 d before surgery[79]
Tofacitinib and baricitinib (Janus kinase inhibitor)	Inhibits heterodimers containing JAK1 or JAK3, resulting in inhibition of IL-2, IL-4, IL-7, IL-9, IL-15, and IL-21[78]	Discontinue 7 d before surgery[79]

Abbreviations: DMARD, disease-modifying antirheumatic drug; IL, interleukin; JAK, Janus kinase; RA, rheumatoid arthritis; TNF, tumor necrosis factor.

Data from Goodman SM, Springer B, Guyatt G, et al. 2017 American College of Rheumatology/ American Association of Hip and Knee Surgeons guideline for the perioperative management of antirheumatic medication in patients with rheumatic diseases undergoing elective total hip or to- tal knee arthroplasty. Arthritis Care Res (Hoboken) 2017;69(8):1111–24; with permission.

avoid hematoma formation. Meticulous wound closure should be emphasized in pa- tients with RA with care taken to produce good skin coaptation while avoiding skin inversion with closure. This will go a long way to decrease the likelihood of postoper- ative wound complications.

Vascular Disease

Vascular compromise is recognized as a potential risk in the patient with RA. This is due to 2 primary considerations. First, patients with RA are at an increased risk for other comorbidities such as vasculitis, vasospasm, or Raynaud disease. In these pa- tients, applying ice to surgical sites postoperatively should be avoided.[64] Second, in the case of rheumatoid forefoot surgery, the deformity is usually long-standing.

Patients should be monitored postoperatively for vascular compromise following surgical correction, as the tension on the soft tissues may result in ischemia[64]; this is especially true when severe, long-standing deformities are corrected.

Neurologic Complications

Patients with RA may present with various neurologic conditions secondary to the disease process. Entrapment neuropathy and peripheral neuropathy (both idiopathic and secondary to medication) are common. Assessment of these conditions should be performed preoperatively to determine if adjunctive surgical procedures should be required at the time of surgery, as an example, a tarsal tunnel release before a lateralizing calcaneal slide osteotomy.[64]

Venous Thromboembolism Prophylaxis

Venous thromboembolism (VTE) events, particularly deep vein thrombosis (DVT) and pulmonary embolism, are troublesome complications. Overall, patients with RA have been observed to have an increased risk in the literature.[68,69] In a meta-analysis of VTE risk among patients with RA, Chung and colleagues[69] found an RA-associated VTE had an increased incidence of 2.18%. However, when assessing patients 1-year postoperatively, no increased risk of hospitalization was observed, suggesting the standard-of-care prophylaxis of patients with RA is adequate.[68,69]

Postoperative considerations

Careful postoperative evaluation of patients with RA should be performed to decrease the risks of complications, particularly among patients with RA with long-standing disease.[64] Patient education is also paramount in minimizing postoperative complications, as infection, wound healing complications, and DVT are all increased risks and should be monitored carefully.[68,69] Functional status of the patient with RA also should be performed. Physical therapy should be considered to assist in rehabilitating the functional stability of the patient during the postoperative course.[64] It is important that patients understand their physical limitations and expectations following surgery, as well as potential complications that may require additional treatment or surgery. A multidisciplinary approach to patient care should be continued during the postoperative period, especially when resuming DMARDs and other RA medications. Increased risks of infection, wound dehiscence, DVT, and other postoperative complications are potential complications in the patient with RA.[35]

SUMMARY

In summary, a thorough perioperative assessment of the patient with RA is important in achieving favorable outcomes. A complete history and physical examination with the appropriate laboratory assessment should be performed, noting deficits and functional limitations secondary to the disease process and concomitant comorbidities. Patients should be educated on the potential risks of surgery, including increased risk of infection, wound healing, and VTE events, as well as underlying cardiovascular, pulmonary, and neurologic impediments that may be complicated by surgery. Management of DMARD medications preoperatively should be in accordance with ACR guidelines at the discretion of the rheumatologist. Discussing postoperative limitations and expectations with the patient before surgery is necessary. Perioperative management of the patient with RA can be challenging; however, collaboration between the surgeon and multidisciplinary team can lead to favorable outcomes.

REFERENCES

1. Mandell BF. Perioperative management of the patient with arthritis or systemic autoimmune disease. In medical management of the surgical patient. Elsevier Inc; 2008. p. 633–55.
2. Gualtierotti R, Parisi M, Ingegnoli F. Perioperative management of patients with inflammatory rheumatic diseases undergoing major orthopaedic surgery: a practical overview. Adv Ther 2018;35(4):439–56.
3. Sharif K, Sharif A, Jumah F, et al. Rheumatoid arthritis in review: clinical, anatomical, cellular and molecular points of view. Clin Anat 2018;31(2):216–23.
4. Bissar L, Almoallim H, Albazli K, et al. Perioperative management of patients with rheumatic diseases. Open Rheumatol J 2013;7:42.
5. Goodman SM, Springer B, Guyatt G, et al. 2017 American College of Rheumatology/American Association of Hip and Knee Surgeons guideline for the perioperative management of antirheumatic medication in patients with rheumatic diseases undergoing elective total hip or total knee arthroplasty. Arthritis Care Res 2017;69(8):1111–24.
6. Cader MZ, Filer A, Hazlehurst J, et al. Performance of the 2010 ACR/EULAR criteria for rheumatoid arthritis: comparison with 1987 ACR criteria in a very early synovitis cohort. Ann Rheum Dis 2011;70(6):949–55.
7. Anderson J, Caplan L, Yazdany J, et al. Rheumatoid arthritis disease activity measures: American College of Rheumatology recommendations for use in clinical practice. Arthritis Care Res 2012;64(5):640–7.
8. Lillegraven S, Prince FH, Shadick NA, et al. Remission and radiographic outcome in rheumatoid arthritis: application of the 2011 ACR/EULAR remission criteria in an observational cohort. Ann Rheum Dis 2012;71(5):681–6.
9. Singh JA, Saag KG, Bridges SL Jr, et al. 2015 American College of Rheumatology guideline for the treatment of rheumatoid arthritis. Arthritis Rheumatol 2016;68(1): 1–26.
10. Kannel WB, Abbott RD. Incidence and prognosis of unrecognized myocardial infarction: an update on the Framingham study. N Engl J Med 1984;311(18): 1144–7.
11. Silvestri L, Maffessanti M, Gregori D, et al. Usefulness of routine pre-operative chest radiography for anaesthetic management: a prospective multicentre pilot study. Eur J Anaesthesiol 1999;11:749–60.
12. Lee TH, Marcantonio ER, Mangione CM, et al. Derivation and prospective validation of a simple index for prediction of cardiac risk of major noncardiac surgery. Circulation 1999;100(10):1043–9.
13. Bushnell BD, Horton KJ, McDonald MF, et al. Perioperative medical comorbidities in the orthopaedic patient. J Am Acad Orthop Surg 2008;16(4):216–27.
14. Nguyen HV, Ludwig SC, Silber J, et al. Rheumatoid arthritis of the cervical spine. Spine J 2004;4(3):329–34.
15. Macarthur A, Kleiman S. Rheumatoid cervical joint disease—a challenge to the anaesthetist. Can J Anaesth 1993;40(2):154–9.
16. Reiter MF, Boden SD. Inflammatory disorders of the cervical spine. Spine (Phila Pa 1976) 1998;23(24):2755–66.
17. Collins DN, Barnes CL, FitzRandolph RL. Cervical spine instability in rheumatoid patients having total hip or knee arthroplasty. Clin Orthop Relat Res 1991;(272): 127–35.
18. Pellicci PM, Ranawat CS, Tsairis P, et al. A prospective study of the progression of rheumatoid arthritis of the cervical spine. J Bone Joint Surg Am 1981;63(3):342–50.

19. Crockard A, Grob D. Rheumatoid arthritis, upper cervical involvement. In: Clark CR, editor. The cervical spine. Philadelphia: JB Lippincott; 1998. p. 705–19.
20. Kolman J, Morris I. Cricoarytenoid arthritis: a cause of acute upper airway obstruction in rheumatoid arthritis. Can J Anaesth 2002;49(7):729–32.
21. Aviña-Zubieta JA, Choi HK, Sadatsafavi M, et al. Risk of cardiovascular mortality in patients with rheumatoid arthritis: a meta-analysis of observational studies. Arthritis Care Res 2008;59(12):1690–7.
22. Liang KP, Myasoedova E, Crowson CS, et al. Increased prevalence of diastolic dysfunction in rheumatoid arthritis. Ann Rheum Dis 2010;69(9):1665–70.
23. Roubille C, Richer V, Starnino T, et al. The effects of tumour necrosis factor inhibitors, methotrexate, non-steroidal anti-inflammatory drugs and corticosteroids on cardiovascular events in rheumatoid arthritis, psoriasis and psoriatic arthritis: a systematic review and meta-analysis. Ann Rheum Dis 2015;74(3):480–9.
24. Maradit-Kremers H, Nicola PJ, Crowson CS, et al. Cardiovascular death in rheumatoid arthritis: a population-based study. Arthritis Rheum 2005;52(3):722–32.
25. Biskup M, Biskup W, Majdan M, et al. Cardiovascular system changes in rheumatoid arthritis patients with continued low disease activity. Rheumatol Int 2018; 38(7):1207–15.
26. Agca R, Heslinga SC, Rollefstad S, et al. EULAR recommendations for cardiovascular disease risk management in patients with rheumatoid arthritis and other forms of inflammatory joint disorders: 2015/2016 update. Ann Rheum Dis 2016; 76(1):17–28.
27. Lake F, Proudman S. Rheumatoid arthritis and lung disease: from mechanisms to a practical approach. Semin Respir Crit Care Med 2014;35(02):222–38. Thieme Medical Publishers.
28. Mori S, Koga Y, Sugimoto M. Different risk factors between interstitial lung disease and airway disease in rheumatoid arthritis. Respir Med 2012;106(11): 1591–9.
29. Roubille C, Haraoui B. Interstitial lung diseases induced or exacerbated by DMARDS and biologic agents in rheumatoid arthritis: a systematic literature review. Semin Arthritis Rheum 2014;43(5):613–26. WB Saunders.
30. Ruderman EM. Overview of safety of non-biologic and biologic DMARDs. Rheumatology 2012;51(suppl_6):vi37–43.
31. Upchurch KS, Kay J. Evolution of treatment for rheumatoid arthritis. Rheumatology 2012;51(suppl_6):vi28–36.
32. Atzeni F, Boiardi L, Sallì S, et al. Lung involvement and drug-induced lung disease in patients with rheumatoid arthritis. Expert Rev Clin Immunol 2013;9(7): 649–57.
33. Diaper R, Wong E, Metcalfe SA. The implications of biologic therapy for elective foot and ankle surgery in patients with rheumatoid arthritis. Foot (Edinb) 2017;30:53–8.
34. Shourt CA, Crowson CS, Gabriel SE, et al. Orthopedic surgery among patients with rheumatoid arthritis 1980-2007: a population-based study focused on surgery rates, sex, and mortality. J Rheumatol 2012;39(3):481–5.
35. Smolen JS, Landewé R, Bijlsma J, et al. EULAR recommendations for the management of rheumatoid arthritis with synthetic and biological disease-modifying antirheumatic drugs: 2016 update. Ann Rheum Dis 2017;76(6):960–77.
36. Fleury G, Mania S, Hannouche D, et al. The perioperative use of synthetic and biological disease-modifying antirheumatic drugs in patients with rheumatoid arthritis. Swiss Med Wkly 2017;147:w14563.
37. Tian H, Cronstein BN. Understanding the mechanisms of action of methotrexate. Bull NYU Hosp Jt Dis 2007;65(3):168–73.

38. Wessels JA, Kooloos WM, De Jonge R, et al. Relationship between genetic variants in the adenosine pathway and outcome of methotrexate treatment in patients with recent-onset rheumatoid arthritis. Arthritis Rheum 2006;54(9):2830–9.
39. Saleh MM, Irshaid YM, Mustafa KN. Methylene tetrahydrofolate reductase genotypes frequencies: association with toxicity and response to methotrexate in rheumatoid arthritis patients. Int J Clin Pharmacol Ther 2015;53(2):154–62.
40. Goodman SM. Rheumatoid arthritis: perioperative management of biologics and DMARDs. Semin Arthritis Rheum 2015;44(6):627–32. WB Saunders.
41. Grennan DM, Gray J, Loudon J, et al. Methotrexate and early postoperative complications in patients with rheumatoid arthritis undergoing elective orthopaedic surgery. Ann Rheum Dis 2001;60(3):214–7.
42. Sany J, Anaya JM, Canovas F, et al. Influence of methotrexate on the frequency of postoperative infectious complications in patients with rheumatoid arthritis. J Rheumatol 1993;20(7):1129–32.
43. Minaur NJ, Kounali D, Vedi S, et al. Methotrexate in the treatment of rheumatoid arthritis. II. In vivo effects on bone mineral density. Rheumatology 2002;41(7):741–9.
44. Uehara R, Suzuki Y, Ichikawa Y. Methotrexate (MTX) inhibits osteoblastic differentiation in vitro: possible mechanism of MTX osteopathy. J Rheumatol 2001;28(2):251–6.
45. Annussek T, Kleinheinz J, Thomas S, et al. Short time administration of antirheumatic drugs—methotrexate as a strong inhibitor of osteoblast's proliferation in vitro. Head Face Med 2012;8(1):26.
46. Smolen JS. Efficacy and safety of the new DMARD leflunomide: comparison to placebo and sulfasalazine in active rheumatoid arthritis. Scand J Rheumatol 1999;28(112):15–21.
47. Smedegård G, Björk J. Sulphasalazine: mechanism of action in rheumatoid arthritis. Rheumatology 1995;34(suppl_2):7–15.
48. Wiese MD, Alotaibi N, O'doherty C, et al. Pharmacogenomics of NAT2 and ABCG2 influence the toxicity and efficacy of sulphasalazine containing DMARD regimens in early rheumatoid arthritis. Pharmacogenomics J 2014;14(4):350.
49. Box SA, Pullar T. Sulphasalazine in the treatment of rheumatoid arthritis. Br J Rheumatol 1997;36(3):382–6.
50. Lafyatis R, York M, Marshak-Rothstein A. Antimalarial agents: closing the gate on toll-like receptors? Arthritis Rheum 2006;54(10):3068–70.
51. Rempenault C, Combe B, Barnetche T, et al. Metabolic and cardiovascular benefits of hydroxychloroquine in patients with rheumatoid arthritis: a systematic review and meta-analysis. Ann Rheum Dis 2018;77(1):98–103.
52. Panek JJ, Jezierska A, Mierzwicki K, et al. Molecular modeling study of leflunomide and its active metabolite analogues. J Chem Inf Model 2005;45(1):39–48.
53. Strand V, Cohen S, Schiff M, et al. Treatment of active rheumatoid arthritis with leflunomide compared with placebo and methotrexate. Arch Intern Med 1999;159(21):2542–50.
54. Fox R, Helfgott SM. Pharmacology, dosing, and adverse effects of leflunomide in the treatment of rheumatoid arthritis. In: Romain PL, editor. UpToDate. Available at: https://www.uptodate.com/contents/pharmacology-dosing-and-adverse-effects-of-leflunomide-in-the-treatment-of-rheumatoid-arthritis. Accessed July 16, 2018.
55. Howe CR, Gardner GC, Kadel NJ. Perioperative medication management for the patient with rheumatoid arthritis. J Am Acad Orthop Surg 2006;14(9):544–51.
56. Fuerst M, Möhl H, Baumgärtel K, et al. Leflunomide increases the risk of early healing complications in patients with rheumatoid arthritis undergoing elective orthopedic surgery. Rheumatol Int 2006;26(12):1138–42.

57. Palmowski Y, Buttgereit T, Dejaco C, et al. "Official View" on glucocorticoids in rheumatoid arthritis: a systematic review of international guidelines and consensus statements. Arthritis Care Res 2017;69(8):1134–41.
58. Somayaji R, Barnabe C, Martin L. Risk factors for infection following total joint arthroplasty in rheumatoid arthritis. Open Rheumatol J 2013;7:119.
59. Saag KG, Shane E, Boonen S, et al. Teriparatide or alendronate in glucocorticoid-induced osteoporosis. N Engl J Med 2007;357(20):2028–39.
60. Saag KG, Zanchetta JR, Devogelaer JP, et al. Effects of teriparatide versus alendronate for treating glucocorticoid-induced osteoporosis: thirty-six–month results of a randomized, double-blind, controlled trial. Arthritis Rheum 2009;60(11): 3346–55.
61. Clement ND, Breusch SJ, Biant LC. Lower limb joint replacement in rheumatoid arthritis. J Orthop Surg Res 2012;7(1):27.
62. Pieringer H, Stuby U, Biesenbach G. Patients with rheumatoid arthritis undergoing surgery: how should we deal with antirheumatic treatment? Semin Arthritis Rheum 2007;36(5):278–86. WB Saunders.
63. Brooks F, Hariharan K. The rheumatoid forefoot. Curr Rev Musculoskelet Med 2013;6(4):320–7.
64. Jacobs AM. Perioperative management of the patient with rheumatoid arthritis. Clin Podiatr Med Surg 2010;27(2):235–42.
65. Bibbo C, Anderson RB, Davis WH. Injury characteristics and the clinical outcome of subtalar dislocations: a clinical and radiographic analysis of 25 cases. Foot Ankle Int 2003;24(2):158–63.
66. Reize P, Leichtle CI, Leichtle UG, et al. Long-term results after metatarsal head resection in the treatment of rheumatoid arthritis. Foot Ankle Int 2006;27(8): 586–90.
67. Anderson T, Rydholm U, Besjakov J, et al. Tibiotalocalcaneal fusion using retrograde intramedullary nails as a salvage procedure for failed total ankle prostheses in rheumatoid arthritis: a report on sixteen cases. Foot Ankle Surg 2005;11(3): 143–7.
68. Goodman SM, Figgie MA. Arthroplasty in patients with established rheumatoid arthritis (RA): mitigating risks and optimizing outcomes. Best Pract Res Clin Rheumatol 2015;29(4–5):628–42.
69. Chung WS, Peng CL, Lin CL, et al. Rheumatoid arthritis increases the risk of deep vein thrombosis and pulmonary thromboembolism: a nationwide cohort study. Ann Rheum Dis 2013;73(10):1774–80.
70. Nguyen DX, Ehrenstein MR. Anti-TNF drives regulatory T cell expansion by paradoxically promoting membrane TNF–TNF-RII binding in rheumatoid arthritis. J Exp Med 2016;213(7):1241–53.
71. Perdriger A. Infliximab in the treatment of rheumatoid arthritis. Biologics 2009;3: 183–91.
72. Michelon MA, Gottlieb AB. Role of golimumab, a TNF-alpha inhibitor, in the treatment of the psoriatic arthritis. Clin Cosmet Investig Dermatol 2010;3:79.
73. Goel N, Stephens S. Certolizumab pegol. MAbs 2010;2(2):137–47. Taylor & Francis.
74. Goldenberg MM. Etanercept, a novel drug for the treatment of patients with severe, active rheumatoid arthritis. Clin Ther 1999;21(1):75–87.
75. Herrero-Beaumont G, Calatrava MJM, Castañeda S. Abatacept mechanism of action: concordance with its clinical profile. Reumatol Clin 2012;8(2):78–83.

76. Buch MH, Smolen JS, Betteridge N, et al. Updated consensus statement on the use of rituximab in patients with rheumatoid arthritis. Ann Rheum Dis 2011;70(6): 909–20.
77. Jones G, Sebba A, Gu J, et al. Comparison of tocilizumab monotherapy versus methotrexate monotherapy in patients with moderate to severe rheumatoid arthritis: the AMBITION study. Ann Rheum Dis 2009;69(1):88–96.
78. Wollenhaupt J, Silverfield J, Lee EB, et al. Safety and efficacy of tofacitinib, an oral janus kinase inhibitor, for the treatment of rheumatoid arthritis in open-label, long-term extension studies. J Rheumatol 2014;41(5):837–52.
79. Franco AS, Iuamoto LR, Pereira RMR. Perioperative management of drugs commonly used in patients with rheumatic diseases: a review. Clinics (Sao Paulo) 2017;72(6):386–90.

Perioperative Understanding of Geriatric Patients

Paris Payton, DPM*, Jeffrey E. Shook, DPM

KEYWORDS

- Geriatric • Dementia • Frailty • Postoperative delirium • Cognitive dysfunction
- Functional dependence • Fall prevention • Transition of care

KEY POINTS

- Developing a strategy for the evaluation of issues affecting the elderly in the perioperative time frame is essential, as this group of patients will soon be the largest segment of patients undergoing surgery.
- Setting reasonable goals for any surgical procedure is important in the elderly patient population. Succinctly conferring these goals to patients, patients' families, and/or caregivers assists in avoiding complications and realizing these surgical goals.
- Assessment of ability to perform activities of daily living preoperatively and gait training/evaluation is mandatory in many elderly patients, especially if a particular patient lives alone.
- Disposition planning or transitional care is more important in this patient population than in any other, and the timely completion of this process cannot be overemphasized.
- A multidisciplinary team approach should be used when considering perioperative issues in elderly patients.

INTRODUCTION

Advances in surgical and anesthetic techniques combined with sophisticated perioperative monitoring are factors that have contributed to an expanding number of older adults undergoing surgery. Individuals older than 65 years represent the fastest growing segment of the population[1,2] and account for more than 40% of all surgical procedures.[3] Patients 65 years of age or older are projected to double to 89 million people between 2010 and 2050,[4] and by the year 2020 elderly adults will be the largest segment of the surgical population.[5] Although age alone cannot adequately predict

Disclosure Statements: The authors have nothing to disclose.
Department of Podiatric Surgery, St. Vincent Charity Medical Center, 2351 East 22nd Street, Cleveland, OH 44115, USA
* Corresponding author.
E-mail address: PPaytonDPM@gmail.com

Clin Podiatr Med Surg 36 (2019) 131–140
https://doi.org/10.1016/j.cpm.2018.08.006
podiatric.theclinics.com

operative outcomes,[6–8] seniors are at higher risk of operative morbidity and mortality.[9,10] A variety of problems are associated with the evaluation and treatment of geriatric patients for podiatric surgery, as older individuals often have multiple comorbid conditions that limit their functional capacity and recovery as well as increase their risk of problems, even death, postoperatively. Decreased functional status, balance problems, the presence of vascular disease and neurologic disorders or deficits coupled with osteopenia as well as cutaneous and connective tissue changes may complicate surgical procedures. Cognitive decline, functional dependence, poor nutrition status, and limited home support may also complicate postoperative recovery.

UNDERSTANDING THE GOALS OF TREATMENT

A clear understanding of the surgical goals in any geriatric patient must be achieved between the podiatrist and patient, family members, and/or caregivers. Discussions with patients and their families or caregivers in regard to preferred treatment and the associated goals of treatment should be comprehensive and thoroughly documented. Careful consideration must be given to preoperative fasting considerations as well as a review of the patients' comorbid conditions and their current medication regimen. Efforts to avoid cognitive and functional decline following surgery should be of utmost importance. Because patients will be undergoing foot or ankle surgery, interference with normal or already compromised ambulation may present a significant risk to geriatric patients. A review of the patients' living conditions and the availability of assistance from family, friends, or agencies should be established. Consideration should also be given to ambulatory status or physical limitations of patients before and following surgery. In this regard, a physical therapy consult preoperatively may help stratify elderly patients' ambulatory capacity before surgery and assist in predicting what will be necessary for the same patients to be able to adequately maneuver after surgery given a particular procedure's effect on postoperative disposition. Physical therapy should assess strength and function of the both the upper and lower extremities.

AGE-RELATED PERIOPERATIVE RISK FACTORS

Older adult surgical patients often require a different level of care than younger patients during the perioperative period. Many have multiple chronic illnesses other than the one for which surgery is required; therefore, they are prone to developing postoperative complications, functional decline, loss of independence, impaired cognition, and other untoward outcomes. However, when age and severity of illness are directly compared, severity of illness is a much better predictor of outcome compared with age. It is essential that patients be assessed individually without being categorized by age, and any factors associated with increased risk of postoperative sequelae and complications should be identified and addressed. The significant patient-associated risk factors in elderly patients that correlate with postoperative adverse outcomes include issues of cognitive impairment and postoperative delirium, frailty, immobility and functional dependence, malnutrition, and the challenges of transitions throughout care.

COGNITIVE IMPAIRMENT AND POSTOPERATIVE DELIRIUM

Cognitive decline and memory dysfunction is a leading cause of functional impairment in the elderly population at large. In 2002, the prevalence of dementia and cognitive impairment without dementia in Americans 71 years of age and older was reported as 13.9% and 22.3%, respectively.[11,12] Cognitive impairment is a problem that increases with age and becomes heightened with hospitalization for critical illness and surgery.[13] Delirium is among the most significant age-related postoperative complications and is characterized by an acute decline in cognitive function and attentiveness developing once hospitalized or after surgery.[14] Behaviors range from placid inactivity to frank agitation and involve varying severities of disorganized thinking and altered consciousness. Although generally a transient phenomenon, delirium is associated with increased mortality,[15] higher costs,[16] and prolonged hospitalization.[17] In elective noncardiac, nonorthopedic surgery, the reported incidence of postoperative delirium is 9%; this incidence increases to 41% after orthopedic procedures.[18] Risk factors include age greater than 65 years, cognitive decline or dementia before surgery, poor vision or hearing, and severe illness. Patients may demonstrate an acute and fluctuating course of dementia with obvious decline from baseline mental status. The inability of patients to focus attention, altered level of consciousness, or disorganized thinking may also be manifestations of delirium. Considerations should be given to uncontrolled pain, hypoxia, infection, medication effect, hypoglycemia, urinary retention, fecal impaction, or any combination thereof.

As compared with postoperative delirium, postoperative cognitive dysfunction is a more subtle but prolonged alteration in cognition,[19] which may involve a range of impairments, including memory, mood, consciousness, and circadian rhythm often manifested by a severe disturbance in the normal sleep-wake cycle.[20] As with delirium, postoperative cognitive dysfunction is associated with longer hospitalizations and higher mortality.[21] Furthermore, there seem to be prolonged, even permanent, consequences with several studies demonstrating cognitive difficulties for months and even years after surgery.[22–24] Lundstom and colleagues[25] found that elderly patients undergoing emergent surgical repair of a fractured hip experienced a 37% rate of significant postoperative cognitive dysfunction among the nondemented fraction of this cohort. They also found that among the patients who experience delirium after surgery, 69% developed frank dementia over a 5-year postoperative follow-up period. There are additional implications, as patients with postoperative cognitive dysfunction at discharge seem more likely to die within a year of surgery.[26]

The American College of Surgeons' (ACS) National Surgical Quality Improvement Program (NSQIP) and the American Geriatrics Society[27] recommend that health care professionals caring for surgical patients should perform an assessment of delirium risk factors, including age greater than 65 years, chronic cognitive decline or dementia, poor vision or hearing, severe illness, and the presence of infection before surgical intervention. They also recommend that all adults identified as high risk for postoperative cognitive dysfunction require regular assessment for delirium by an appropriate health care team member using a validated screening instrument or measure. These health care professionals should also evaluate all postoperative patients demonstrating delirium for possible precipitating conditions, such as uncontrolled pain, hypoxia, pneumonia, infection, electrolyte abnormalities, urinary retention, fecal impaction, mind-altering medications, and hypoglycemia. The first step in management is to investigate possible causes. After addressing underlying causes, it is recommended that health care professionals treat older adults displaying delirium with multicomponent nonpharmacologic interventions, reserving pharmacologic therapies for patients who pose a threat to themselves or others with agitated, hyperactive delirium behaviors.[27] The best treatment of delirium is prevention, and current evidence shows that 30% to 40% of postoperative delirium cases are preventable.[28]

FRAILTY

Frailty is generally defined as a state of weakness and susceptibility to stress arising from low physiologic reserve that is not necessarily defined or constrained by age or presence of comorbidities.[29] Relevant characteristics include such age-associated declines in lean body mass, strength, endurance, balance, ambulatory ability, and lowered activity levels. Multiple components must be present in order to constitute frailty. Frailty has emerged as an important predictor of operative risk among elderly surgical patients, and measuring frailty before surgery in older adults may confer added risk stratification beyond age and traditional perioperative risk factors. A simple, useful frailty scale has been developed that assists in the identification and characterization of such patients.[30] The scale uses a 4-level classification across the spectrum of fitness to frailty as outlined next:

1. Able to ambulate without assistance and perform activities of daily living (ADLs), continent, no cognitive impairment
2. Bladder incontinence only, no assistance needed and no cognitive impairment
3. One or more instances of needing assistance with mobility or ADLs, has cognitive impairment (but not dementia), or has bowel/bladder incontinence
4. Two or more instances of being totally dependent for transfers or one or more ADLs or bowel/bladder incontinence and a diagnosis of dementia

This syndrome of frailty results in a progressive decline in overall function, loss of physiologic reserve, and increased vulnerability to disease and death. In addition, frailty predisposes these patients to falls, disability, social isolation, and the need for institutionalization.[31] However, younger individuals can overcome health challenges because of adequate physiologic reserves conferred by their youth and overall better health. In aging, greater proportions of physiologic reserve are directed to maintaining basic bodily homeostasis, leaving less capacity to address health challenges and stress. Thus, the physiologic stress associated with surgery can present increasingly higher states of vulnerability in elderly patients resulting in increasing levels of frailty.[31]

FALL PREVENTION

Elderly patients are at increased risk of falls, and it has been reported that more than 30% of people aged 65 years and older sustain at least one fall annually.[32] This population is at even greater fall risk following orthopedic and podiatric surgery as a result of altered weight-bearing status, mobility assistance, and postoperative dressings. Geriatric patients undergoing surgery should be evaluated for fall risk factors before surgery. These risk factors include preoperative impaired gait and mobility, the effects of pain medications, as well as the effects of other medications, such as antihypertensives or diuretics. Evaluation of patients for fall risks may include the Morse fall risk scale, which includes assessment for history of falling, medical diagnoses increasing fall risk, mental status, the use of ambulatory aids, and other impediments to ambulation. Altered mental state may increase the predisposition of patients to falls following surgery, and this should be taken into consideration if any postoperative cognitive dysfunction presents following surgery. Inquiry should be made regarding the home environment, such as the location of the bathroom, stairs, or other obstructions to ambulation. The presence of neuropathy, visual impairment, dehydration, and the need for frequent urination should be considered. If it is anticipated that an elderly patient will be significantly impeded in ambulation following surgery, a discussion should be held with the family members or caretakers regarding efforts at fall prevention.

POOR NUTRITION

Increasing age is associated with a poor nutrition status because of decreased access to wholesome food and inadequate food intake, reduced appetite, poor dentition, chronic diseases, medications, changes in metabolism, and physiologic issues. Nutritional deficits are common in the elderly and have been reported to occur in as many as 38.7% of hospitalized geriatric patients.[33] Such patients should be identified immediately on admission so that proper nutritional supplementation can be initiated as soon as possible. Malnutrition is not only frequently found among elderly patients but it has also been identified as an independent risk factor for morbidity, mortality, and the length of hospitalization. In a prospective study of 100 patients undergoing major abdominal surgery conducted by Sungurtekin and colleagues,[34] they found that higher mortality was reported for the malnourished group, whereas no mortality was reported in the well-nourished group. Another study conducted by Kuzu and colleagues[35] looking at 460 patients (mean age 55.3 years) undergoing major elective surgery reported that morbidity, particularly in the case of severe infection, was significantly higher among malnourished patients, with the odds ratio for morbidity ranging from 2.3 to 3.47 in well-nourished versus malnourished patients.

Serum albumin and prealbumin have long been effective and cheap measurements for nutrition status in surgical patients. There is controversy surrounding the utility of albumin as a marker of nutritional status; however, preoperative albumin levels have been shown to predict postoperative outcomes. In a study of more than 87,000 major noncardiac operations, Khuri and colleagues[36] assessed perioperative risk using 67 variables. They found 44 variables to be significant in predicting 30-day postoperative mortality. Of these variables, serum albumin was the more important predictor of 30-day mortality. In another study by Arozullah and colleagues,[37] they reported age, low albumin, and low functional status as risk factors for postoperative respiratory failure. Further, in a systematic review of 15 articles on nutritional status and postoperative complications, van Stijn and colleagues[38] reported that only weight loss of 10% or greater in the previous 6 months and low serum albumin were significant predictors of postoperative outcomes after general surgery.

Prealbumin, another hepatic protein known to reflect nutritional status, has some benefits over albumin in assessing nutrition in the perioperative setting. First, prealbumin has a shorter half-life of 2 days as compared with the 20-day half-life of albumin,[39] making it a better indicator of acute changes in nutritional status. Second, because prealbumin is unaffected by hydration status, it may be a more reliable marker of nourishment than albumin, particularly in patients who have greater fluid fluctuations[40] (eg, renal patients, congestive heart failure [CHF]). In a prospective cohort study of 114 patients undergoing cytoreduction surgery for ovarian cancer, Geisler and colleagues[41] reported that low prealbumin (<10 mg/dL) was associated with increased complications and mortality. In a retrospective study of 641 consecutive patients who underwent surgery for gastrointestinal malignancy, Lin and colleagues[39] reported that low prealbumin levels (<18 mg/dL) predicted overall morbidity and infectious complications.

As a result of the physiologic stress response brought about by physical trauma, the nutrient needs of trauma patients presenting for orthopedic surgery may be greatly increased. Caloric needs postoperatively can be as high as twice the normal amount required for weight maintenance and the support of basic physical functioning. The greatly increased needs for protein and calories to support healing postoperatively are often difficult for patients to achieve, and supplementation should be implemented as necessary. Furthermore, the perioperative fasting regimen may result in a negative net nutrient balance in geriatric patients; appropriate adjustments should be made leading up to surgery. Typically, patients are instructed to remain at nothing-by-mouth status following midnight before the day of surgery. However, the impact of a nothing-by-mouth status may be more significant in geriatric patients; no association has been demonstrated between a shortened clear fluid fast (2–3 hours before surgery) and postoperative complications. The ASA's current guidelines for nonemergent surgery[27] indicate that clear fluids (eg, water, fruit juices without pulp, carbonated beverages, clear tea, and black coffee) may be taken up to 2 hours before elective procedures requiring general anesthesia, regional anesthesia, or sedation/analgesia. Adults scheduled for an elective nonemergent surgical procedure should fast from a light meal and/or nonhuman milk for at least 6 hours. Additional fasting (8 hours or more) may be required depending on the type of food ingested, comorbidities/diseases, or other areas that may affect gastric emptying or fluid volumes.[27]

As further specified by the ACS' NSQIP and the American Geriatrics Society,[27] older adult patients should undergo daily evaluation of their ability to take in adequate nutrition, including risk of aspiration. It is also recommended that elderly surgical patients should be sitting upright while eating and for 1 hour postprandial. The health care team should make every effort to initiate normal food intake or enteral feeding as early as possible, and adequate hydration should be implemented and monitored for at least 5 days following surgery. There should be an initiation of dietary consultation and/or formal swallowing assessment if indicated. Patients with signs of dysphagia, which include coughing or choking with swallowing; difficulty initiating swallow; drooling; change in dietary habits, voice, or speech; nasal regurgitation; and history of aspiration pneumonia, should undergo a formal swallowing assessment.[27]

ANTICOAGULATION THERAPY AND DEEP VENOUS THROMBOSIS PROPHYLAXIS

Many geriatric patients are on anticoagulation therapy; discontinuation of these medications may have associated risks, including increased risk of thrombosis, stent occlusion, deep venous thrombosis (DVT), or stroke. A consultation with cardiology or internal medicine should be considered in particular patients, and inquiry should be made in regard to not only the anticoagulant used but what it is being used to treat. Older age is also reported to confer an additional risk for DVT.[42] An estimated 20% to 30% of patients undergoing general surgery without prophylaxis develop DVT; the incidence rate is as high as 40% in those undergoing hip and knee surgery, gynecologic cancer operations, open prostatectomies, and major neurosurgical procedures. Geriatric patients should be stratified regarding the risk for DVT as well as the risks for bleeding. Risk factors for increased incidence of DVT include increasing age, history of cancer, active antineoplastic therapy, prior history of DVT, venous insufficiency, CHF, smoking, anticipated immobility, obesity, or irritable bowel syndrome. Each patient should be evaluated individually for such risk factors.

TRANSITIONS OF CARE

Transitional care refers to interventions that intend to ensure continuity and coordination of care as patients move between health care settings. Older persons who are hospitalized for acute illnesses, including surgical interventions, often lose their independence and are discharged to institutions for short-term or long-term care. A recent study of Medicare beneficiaries found that over the 30-day period following hospital discharge, 60% of patients made a single transfer, 18% 2 transfers, 9% 3 transfers, and 4% 4 or more transfers.[43] This pattern of discontinuity of care is particularly common in the orthopedic and podiatric settings, as the rehabilitative requirement of this population postoperatively is essential to provide physical and occupational therapy.

With increasing pressures to shorten the length of hospital stay, the transfer of patient care from the hospital to community settings can oftentimes be unsystematic, unstandardized, and fragmented. The process is frequently burdened with poor understanding of postoperative recovery and instruction by the patients, because of both low health literacy and poor communication on the part of providers. These challenges and other factors can result in an increased rate of postoperative complications and subsequent hospital readmissions[43]; however, optimal care transitions from the hospital to home or post–acute care settings can help reduce the length and number of hospital stays as well as the utilization of emergency services.[44,45]

Risk factors for unsuccessful transitions of care have been identified, including advanced age, serious illness, and various psychosocial considerations, such as insufficient support and a history of prior hospitalization. Coleman and colleagues[46] published a patient-focused assessment protocol in regard to estimating postoperative outcomes following health care transitions. Specific domains of care used in the Care Transitions Measure (CTM) were developed to enhance quality of care as patients are transferred from one setting to another. The areas measured include the reliability and timeliness of information transfer; the preparation of patients, families, and the caregivers for transfer; the support to ensure successful patient self-management; and the need to empower patients to define and assert their individual goals and preferences of care. Lower scores on the CTM at discharge predict subsequent emergency department visits and repeat hospitalizations.

Specialized acute-care geriatric units have been created and have shown improved patient outcomes without increased costs. Units have environmental enhancements appropriate for older patients, such as improved lighting, contrasting colors, bold patterns, furnishings suited for elderly persons, uncluttered hallways, large clocks and calendars, and handrails. Patient-centered care emphasizes independence, including specific protocols for the rehabilitation and the prevention of disability. The focus is on discharge planning, with the ultimate goal of returning patients to their independence. Medical care is intensely reviewed to minimize the adverse effects of procedures and medications. Regardless of the extent and nature of the systems used, efficient transfer of information remains a key component of successful transition of care and optimal outcomes. Good communication between all parties involved in the care and transition of elderly patients is paramount.

In regard to discharge planning, the ACS' NSQIP and the American Geriatrics Society[27] recommend that the health care team assess patients' social support involving family and/or caregivers in regard to the need for skilled nursing versus home health care on discharge. They also recommend that a discussion with patients and/or their caregivers should be held and documented in regard to the postoperative course, instructions, and medication regimen. Patients should undergo assessments of nutrition, cognition, ambulatory ability, and functional status before discharge; comprehensive discharge instructions should be provided along with follow-up plans as patients transition into rehabilitation.

PHYSICAL THERAPY AND REHABILITATION OF THE ELDERLY

Elderly patients are at an increased risk for developing functional decline during or following hospitalization. Studies have shown that more than 30% of patients older than 65 years develop a new disability pertaining to ADLs during hospitalization; by 1 year, less than half of these patients have recovered to preoperative function levels.[47,48] The stress of surgery further increases the risk of functional decline; postoperative rehabilitation should be aimed to optimize physical, intellectual, psychological, and social function. Following surgery, health care professionals should implement interventions for the prevention of functional decline in the postoperative older adult, including early mobilization and physical therapy.[49] A multidisciplinary approach should be implemented incorporating both physical and occupational therapy with the ultimate goal of age-related complication prevention. Following the initial period of healing, which usually takes approximately 6 to 12 weeks, a physical therapy program should be initiated, which is directed at improving muscle strength, endurance, coordination, and balance. The rehabilitation process should be expected to take 6 to 12 months depending on the procedure performed; expectations of recovery must address the preoperative health of patients, emphasizing that the relative fitness or frailty of patients is more important than their chronologic age.

REFERENCES

1. US Census Bureau Population Division. Annual estimates of resident population by sex, age, race, and Hispanic origin for the United States: April 1, 2010 to July 1, 2012. Washington, DC: Government Printing Office; 2013.
2. US Census Bureau Population Division. Percent distribution of the projected population by selected age groups and sex for the United States: 2015 to 2060 (NP2012-T3L). Washington, DC: Government Printing Office; 2013.
3. National Center for Health Statistics. National hospital discharge survey, 2010. Hyattsville (MD): Public Health Service; 2010.
4. Werner C. The older population: 2010. Washington, DC: U.S. Census Bureau; 2011.
5. Etzioni DA, Liu JH, Maffart MA, et al. The aging population and its impact on the surgery workforce. Ann Surg 2003;238(2):170–7.
6. El-Haddawi F, Abu-Zidan FM, Jones W. Factors affecting surgical outcome in the elderly at Auckland Hospital. ANZ J Surg 2002;72:537–41.
7. Fleisher LA, Beckman JA, Brown KA, et al. ACC/AHA 2007 guidelines on perioperative cardiovascular evaluation and care for noncardiac surgery: executive summary: a report of the American College of Cardiology/American Heart Association Task Force on Practice Guidelines (Writing Committee to Revise the 2002 Guidelines on Perioperative Cardiovascular Evaluation for Noncardiac Surgery): developed in Collaboration with the American Society of Echocardiography, American Society of Nuclear Cardiology, Heart Rhythm Society, Society of Cardiovascular Anesthesiologists, Society for Cardiovascular Angiography and Interventions, Society for Vascular Medicine and Biology, and Society for Vascular Surgery. Circulation 2007;116:1971–96.
8. Sundermann SH, Dademasch A, Seifert B, et al. Frailty is a predictor of short- and mid-term mortality after elective cardiac surgery independently of age. Interact Cardiovasc Thorac Surg 2014;18(5):580–5.
9. Deiner S, Silverstein JH. Anesthesia for geriatric patients. Minerva Anestesiol 2011;77:180–9.
10. Ronning B, Wyller TB, Jordhoy MS, et al. Frailty indicators and functional status in older patients after colorectal cancer surgery. J Geriatr Oncol 2014;5:26–32.
11. Plassman BL, Langa KM, Fisher GG, et al. Prevalence of cognitive impairment without dementia in the United Status. Ann Intern Med 2008;148(6):427–34.
12. Plassman BL, Langa KM, Fisher GG, et al. Prevalence of dementia in the United States: the aging, demographics, and memory study. Neuroepidemiology 2007; 29(1–2):125–32.

13. Ehlenbach WJ, Hough CL, Crane PK, et al. Association between acute care and critical illness hospitalization and cognitive function in older adults. JAMA 2010; 303(8):763–70.
14. Inouye SK, Robinson T, Blaum C, et al. American geriatrics society expert panel on postoperative delirium in older adults. J Am Geriatr Society 2014;63(1): 142–50.
15. Ely EW, Shintani A, Truman B, et al. Delirium as a predictor of mortality in mechanically ventilated patients in the ICU. JAMA 2004;291(14):1753–62.
16. Milbrandt EB, Deppen S, Harrison PL, et al. Costs associated with delirium in mechanically ventilated patients in the ICU. Crit Care Med 2004;32(4):955–62.
17. Ely EW, Gautam S, Margolin R, et al. The impact of delirium in the intensive care unit on hospital length of stay. Intensive Care Med 2001;27(12):1892–900.
18. Dyer CB, Ashton CM, Teasedale TA. Postoperative delirium: a review of 80 primary data-collection studies. Arch Intern Med 1995;155(5):461–5.
19. Terrando N, Brzezinski M, Degos V, et al. Perioperative cognitive decline in the aging population. Mayo Clin Proc 2011;86(9):885–93.
20. Caza N, Taha R, Qi Y, et al. The effects of surgery and anesthesia on memory and cognition. Prog Brain Res 2008;169:409–22.
21. Steinmetz J, Christensen KB, Lund T, et al. Long-term consequences of postoperative cognitive dysfunction. Anesthesiology 2009;110(3):548–55.
22. Moller JT, Cluitmans P, Rasmussen LS, et al. Long-term post-operative dysfunction in the elderly. ISPOCD1 study. ISPOCD investigators. Lancet 1998; 351(9106):857–61.
23. Price CC, Garvan CW, Monk TG. Type and severity of cognitive decline in older adults after noncardiac surgery. Anesthesiology 2008;108(1):8–17.
24. Abildstrom H, Rassmussen LS, Rentowl P, et al. Cognitive dysfunction 1-2 years after non-cardiac surgery in the elderly. ISPOCD group. Acta Anaesthesiol Scand 2000;44(10):1246–51.
25. Lundstom M, Bucht EA, Karlsson S, et al. Dementia after delirium in patient with femoral neck fractures. J Am Geriatr Soc 2003;51:1002–6.
26. Monk TG, Weldon BC, Garvan CW, et al. Predictors of cognitive dysfunction after major noncardiac surgery. Anesthesiology 2008;108(1):18–30.
27. Mohanty S, Rosenthal R, Russell M, et al. Optimal perioperative management of the geriatric patient: a best practices guideline from the American College of Surgeons NSQIP and the American Geriatrics Society. J Am Coll Surg 2016;222(5): 930–47.
28. Siddiqi N, Holt R, Britton AM, et al. Interventions for preventing delirium in hospitalised patients. Cochrane Database Syst Rev 2007;(2):CD005563.
29. Xue QL. The frailty syndrome: definition and natural history. Clin Geriatr Med 2011;27:1–15.
30. Rockwood K, Stadnyk K, MacKnight C, et al. A brief clinical instrument to classify frailty in elderly people. Lancet 1999;353:205–6.
31. MacKenzie CR, Cornell CN, Memtsoudis SG. Perioperative care of the elderly orthopedic patient. Perioperative care of the orthopedic patient. Springer; 2014. p. 209–19.
32. World Health Organization. WHO global report on falls prevention in older age. Geneva (Switzerland: World Health Organization; 2008. Available at: http://www.who.int/iris/handle/10665/43811.
33. Kaiser MJ, Bauer JM, Rämsch C, et al, Mini Nutritional Assessment International Group. Frequency of malnutrition in older adults: a multinational perspective using the mini nutritional assessment. J Am Geriatr Soc 2010;58:1734–8.

34. Sungurtekin H, Sungurtekin U, Balci C, et al. The influence of nutritional status on complications after major intra-abdominal surgery. J Am Coll Nutr 2004;23(3): 227–32.

35. Kuzu MA, Terzioğlu H, Genc V, et al. Preoperative nutritional risk assessment in predicting postoperative outcome in patients undergoing major surgery. World J Surg 2006;30(3):378–90.

36. Khuri SF, Daley J, Henderson W, et al. Risk adjustment of the postoperative mortality rate for the comparative assessment of the quality of surgical care: results of the National Veterans Affairs Surgical Risk Study. J Am Coll Surg 1997;185(4): 315–27.

37. Arozullah AM, Daley J, Henderson WG, et al. Multifactorial risk index for predicting postoperative respiratory failure in men after major noncardiac surgery. The National Veterans Administration Surgical Quality Improvement Program. Ann Surg 2000;232(2):242–53.

38. van Stijn MFM, Korkic-Halilovic I, Bakker MSM, et al. Preoperative nutrition status and postoperative outcome in elderly general surgery patients: a systematic review. JPEN J Parenter Enteral Nutr 2013;37(1):37–43.

39. Lin MY, Liu WY, Tolan AM, et al. Preoperative serum albumin but not prealbumin is an excellent predictor of postoperative complications and mortality in patients with gastrointestinal cancer. Am Surg 2011;77(10):1286–9.

40. Mears E. Outcomes of continuous process improvement of a nutritional care program incorporating serum prealbumin measurements. Nutrition 1996;12(7–8):479–84.

41. Geisler JP, Linnemeier GC, Thomas AJ, et al. Nutritional assessment using prealbumin as an objective criterion to determine whom should not undergo primary radical cytoreductive surgery for ovarian cancer. Gynecol Oncol 2007;106(1):128–31.

42. Seung YL, Du HR, Chin YC, et al. Incidence of deep vein thrombosis after major lower limb orthopedic surgery: analysis of a nationwide claim registry. Yonsei Med J 2015;56(1):139–45.

43. Chugh A, Williams MV, Grigsby J, et al. Better transitions: improving comprehension of discharge instructions. Front Health Serv Manage 2009;25:11–32.

44. Jencks SF, Williams MV, Coleman EA. Rehospitalizations among patients in the Medicare fee-for-service program. N Engl J Med 2009;360:1418–28.

45. Chiu WK, Newcomer R. A systematic review of nurse-assisted case management to improve hospital discharge transition outcomes for the elderly. Prof Case Manag 2007;12:330–6.

46. Coleman EA, Min SJ, Chomiak A, et al. Posthospital care transitions: patterns, complications, and risk identification. Health Serv Res 2004;39(5):1449.

47. Covinsky KE, Palmer RM, Fortinsky RH, et al. Loss of independence in activities of daily living in older adults hospitalized with medical illnesses: increased vulnerability with age. J Am Geriatr Soc 2003;51:451–8.

48. Covinsky KE, Palmer RM, Counsell SR, et al. Functional status before hospitalization in acutely ill older adults: validity and clinical importance of retrospective reports. J Am Geriatr Soc 2000;48:164–9.

49. Orosz GM, Magaziner J, Hannan EL, et al. Association of timing of surgery for hip fracture and patient outcome. JAMA 2004;291(14):1738–43.

Obesity-Related Foot Pain
Diagnosis and Surgical Planning

Jared L. Moon, DPM[a],*, Karen M. Moon, DPM[b],
Dylan M. Carlisle, DPM[b]

KEYWORDS

- Obesity • Management of obesity-related foot pain • Achilles tendonitis
- Plantar fasciitis

KEY POINTS

- Obesity is a significant risk factor for poor surgical outcomes and complications.
- Type 1 obesity-related foot pain should initially be treated conservatively; when surgery is necessary, subtalar joint arthrodesis is a better surgical option than Dwyer osteotomy.
- Type 2 obesity-related foot pain can also usually be treated conservatively; patients in this group usually respond better to treatment. Surgical treatments include tendo Achilles lengthening versus gastrocnemius recession.
- Type 3 obesity-related foot pain can be treated conservatively with custom orthotics, bracing, or nonsteroidal anti-inflammatory drugs. Surgical management consists of arch reconstruction with subtalar joint arthrodesis.

INTRODUCTION

Obesity in combination with foot pathologic condition creates a significant challenge for the foot and ankle surgeon. The World Health Organization Web site estimates that since 1975 worldwide obesity has tripled with 1.9 billion adults being overweight, of which 650 million are obese.[1] Even more concerning is the fact that childhood obesity rates have risen drastically from 4% in 1975 to 18% in 2016.[1] Clearly, this problem is only worsening. The Centers for Disease Control and Prevention (CDC) Web site states that more than one-third of the US population (36.5%) is obese.[2] The CDC also estimated the medical cost of obesity in 2008 to be 147 billion dollars.[2] It is expected that by 2030 more than 50% of adults will be obese.[3] Statistics like these are alarming, yet potentially not that surprising to foot and ankle surgeons as they are dealing with these patient populations on a daily basis. Obesity is a significant

Disclosure Statements: None.
[a] St. Mary Medical Center, 1500 South Lake Park Avenue, Hobart, IN 46342, USA; [b] DeKalb Medical Center, 2701 North Decatur Road, Decatur, GA 30033, USA
* Corresponding author.
E-mail address: Jared.l.moon@gmail.com

Clin Podiatr Med Surg 36 (2019) 141–151
https://doi.org/10.1016/j.cpm.2018.08.008
podiatric.theclinics.com

risk factor for poor surgical outcomes and complications. In this article, the diagnosis of foot pain specific to obesity is discussed, in addition to evaluating how treatment plans both conservative and surgical may need to be modified for obese patients.

DIAGNOSIS OF OBESITY-RELATED FOOT PAIN

The authors believe foot pain caused by obesity is relatively common and presents in predictable patterns. These presentations or predictable patterns, once recognized, oftentimes are appreciated on a daily basis. Symptoms after obesity-related foot pain are often misunderstood leading to failed conservative measures, unwarranted surgery, wrong procedure selection, and, in general, unsuccessful treatment plans. In an attempt to avoid these pitfalls, the process of diagnosis/classification is delineated into 3 types of presentations. Although this classification represents a majority of patients with obesity-related pathologic condition, the astute clinician will recognize outliers exist that do not fall within the following classification scheme.

Type 1 obesity-related foot pain is characterized by pain to the dorsal lateral midfoot area. Often the patient will point to the fifth metatarsal base area, but usually the pain is generalized along the lateral midfoot with extension of pain into either the rearfoot or forefoot. There will be no history of trauma. Radiographs will be negative. MRI is usually negative, although marrow edema or water-weighted pulse sequences may be seen at the lateral midfoot area. Clinical examination will show a neutral heel position with the patient non-weight-bearing with a flexible subtalar joint, although on weight-bearing examination heel varus is seen. Ankle equinus may or may not be present. This foot type is not that different from a flexible cavus foot. On weight-bearing, the patient likely has a heel varus positional deformity that is caused by excessive weight rather than a plantar flexed first ray with or without or neurologic cause. With the heel in the varus position during weight bearing, the lateral foot will be loaded under significant pressure resulting in pain.

Type 2 obesity-related foot pain is distinguished by pain generalized throughout the entire midfoot area. Usually pain is localized to the dorsal midfoot, although plantar midfoot pain presentations can be seen. Type 2 is seen with less frequency than type 1. No history of trauma is present. Radiographs will be negative. MRI will also be negative, but as in type 1 marrow, edema may be seen anywhere throughout the midfoot, which can lead to misdiagnosis of stress fracture. Clinical examinations will show a structurally normal foot. The heel will be in neutral position on weight-bearing with no varus or valgus deformity. Ankle equinus will be present and is likely the contributing factor in causing pain at the midfoot because significant pressure is transferred through this area of the foot during gait.

Type 3 obesity-related foot pain is very similar in presentation to stage 2 posterior tibial tendonitis, whereby a flexible flat foot deformity is seen. It differs from a stage 2 posterior tibial tendon dysfunction in that pain is typically along the plantar medial arch of the foot rather than the posterior tibial tendon. A clinical examination usually shows arch collapse, heel valgus, and equinus. Radiographs show typical findings of a flexible flat foot without arthritic changes. MRI is usually void of any posterior tibial tendon pathologic condition. More than likely these patients have always had a pronated foot type, and as body weight increases, so does severity of arch collapse in turn leading to increased pressure along the medial arch of the foot. In a systematic review on body composition and foot structure, Butterworth and colleagues[4] showed a strong association between obesity and pes planus.

In addition to the above described presentations, it is not unusual to see common foot and ankle pathologic condition such as plantar fasciitis and Achilles tendonitis presenting in combination with obesity. To what level obesity has an effect on these common pathologic conditions remains unknown but needs to be considered. An understanding or appreciation for this will help with appropriate treatment plan as discussed later (**Table 1**).

MANAGEMENT OF OBESITY-RELATED FOOT PAIN

Type 1 obesity-related foot pain should initially be treated conservatively with shoe gear changes, arch supports, anti-inflammatory medication, and limiting activity levels. Walking boots and protected weight-bearing may also be helpful in cases whereby pain is more severe. In addition, diet modifications should be recommended and weight loss encouraged. Lower-body exercise and cardiovascular exercise should be avoided, but upper body strengthening and flexibility-type exercise should be encouraged. In cases whereby pain does not improve, surgical management may be necessary. If the patient is making good progress with weight loss but still having continued foot pain, it is best to hold off on surgery because pain may eventually resolve with significant weight loss. In cases where surgery is needed, it may seem reasonable to address the flexible rearfoot varus deformity with a Dwyer-type osteotomy. One would expect this to neutralize the heel position and help offload pressure on the lateral column of the foot where the patient has pain. In the authors' experience, Dwyer or lateral calcaneal slide osteotomies are inadequate at reducing varus deformity of the heel in obese patients. The inability of this procedure to reduce heel deformity is likely secondary to the large amount of weight being transferred on heel strike. The authors recommend addressing this with subtalar joint arthrodesis placed in a neutral to a slightly pronated position. Heel varus deformity can easily be corrected through subtalar joint arthrodesis, and recurrence of varus deformity with weight bearing is uncommon. The authors realize that the current trend in foot and ankle surgery is to not fuse flexible or nonarthritic joints, but they think this is a situation whereby arthrodesis is necessary.

Management of type 2 obesity-related foot pain is primarily treated with conservative care. Conservative care usually consists of Achilles stretching exercises, shoe gear modifications, orthotics, and anti-inflammatory medication. Discussing diet changes with the patient is also recommended, and upper-body exercise should be encouraged. In the face of failed conservative treatment modalities, surgical management with Achilles lengthening or gastrocnemius recession may be reasonable, although not usually necessary. Type 2 patients seem to respond to conservative treatment plans as compared with type 1 patients. Weight loss needs to be a serious long-term goal for these patients, because they can predictably develop midfoot arthritis over time.

Type 3 obesity-related foot pain is treated very similar to how an adult-acquired flatfoot or posterior tibial tendonitis is treated. Conservative care consists of anti-inflammatory medication, custom orthotics, and advanced bracing. Physical therapy

Table 1		
The 3 types of foot pain, comparing locations of pain, and expected foot structure		
Type	Foot Structure	Location of Pain
1	Flexible heel varus	Dorsal lateral midfoot
2	Neutral heel with ankle equinus	Dorsal midfoot
3	Flexible flatfoot with heel valgus	Plantar medial arch

is only helpful if there is posterior tibial tendonitis, although in the authors' experience usually the tendon has good function and is free of pain with symptoms typically localized to the plantar medial arch. Periods of restricted activity with walking boots may be necessary. Diet modifications should be recommended. Upper-extremity exercise should be encouraged. Surgery may be necessary in some cases. Surgery should focus on arch reconstruction with rearfoot arthrodesis. Usually isolated subtalar joint arthrodesis is adequate. Although this type of flatfoot is usually flexible, the authors advise against osteotomies because reoccurrence of deformity is common secondary to the presence of obesity. Ankle equinus should be addressed when present (**Box 1**).

Management of plantar fasciitis in the obese patient is often very challenging. Standard conservative treatment options should be attempted. An aggressive weight loss plan with diet and exercise should be encouraged. Avoiding surgery is preferred; however, this can be difficult for the patient to accept as plantar fascial pain can be quite severe and debilitating. The authors do not recommend plantar fasciotomy in obese patients for various reasons. Mainly, one would expect obese patients to be at risk for developing significant arch collapse following plantar fasciotomy, effectively giving the patient a foot described above as type 3 obesity-related foot pain. In addition, patients can develop lateral column foot pain following plantar fasciotomy. Obese patients may be at higher risk for developing lateral column foot pain due to increased midfoot and lateral column loading from excess weight, in effect, creating a foot type similar to that described above as type 1 obesity-related foot pain. A reasonable surgical approach may be to address ankle equinus with gastrocnemius recession and avoiding a plantar fasciotomy. An article by Ficke and colleagues[5] has shown gastrocnemius tendon recession to improve foot function in obese patients.

Achilles tendonitis/tendinopathy with posterior heel spur is another common pathologic condition that can be further complicated by obesity. Standard conservative treatment approach should be attempted before surgery with weight loss encouraged. Lymphedema may be present in these cases and is often overlooked. Referral to a lymphedema clinic can be helpful. Proper management of lymphedema can help reduce pain and, if surgery becomes necessary, can make postoperative casting easier. As an isolated procedure, a gastrocnemius recession may provide significant symptomatic relief without the introduction of the attendant complications typically encountered with Achilles detachment and spur resection surgery. Postoperative convalescence following gastrocnemius recession can be simple ambulation in a walking boot without instituting non-weight-bearing with crutches and/or walker. If Achilles detachment and posterior spur resection surgery are contemplated, 3 specific elements of this surgical process should be considered. First, reattachment via advanced anchoring systems should be used in most instances. Second, a gastrocnemius recession should be considered because this allows for more of an anatomic reinsertion of the Achilles without significant tension or loading placed on the Achilles complex. Finally, the addition of a flexor hallucis longus (FHL) tendon transfer may be

Box 1	
Comparison of surgical plans for the 3 types of foot pain	
Type	Surgical Approach Recommended
1	Subtalar joint arthrodesis
2	No surgery/TAL/gastrocnemius recession
3	Subtalar joint arthrodesis
Abbreviation: TAL, tendo achilles lengthening.	

advised depending on amount of diseased Achilles tendon removal. As compared with the nonobese patient, there should be a low threshold to augment the remaining Achilles with the FHL tendon. The added force, due to the obesity, transmitted through the Achilles may not be sustainable over time in a tendon that is diseased and has been debrided. The addition of a FHL tendon transfer may add extra strength and help protect the patient from significant complications in the case of a fall or any misstep that causes excessive dorsiflexion of the ankle. **Fig. 1** shows an example of a difficult to manage complication in an obese patient with a body mass index (BMI) of 45 with a fall 5 weeks postoperatively and rupture of a previously repaired Achilles tendon at the insertion. **Figs. 2** and **3** show revision with FHL transfer and Achilles allograft.

It is not uncommon for obese patients to present with combined symptoms of plantar fasciitis and Achilles tendonitis. Combined inferior and posterior heel pain can be frustrating for both physician and patient, because this can be very difficult to manage. Immediately starting these patients in physical therapy and immobilization in a walking boot can be helpful to sort out which of the 2 conditions is actually causing the pain. With this approach, the pain can be eliminated from at least one of these locations, and then treatment can be refocused on the main area of concern. As with all conditions described above, weight loss needs to be addressed because surgical management of both these conditions at the same time is not ideal. In the situation whereby both conditions need to be addressed surgically, the authors recommend proceeding with caution. In their experience, combined resection of posterior and inferior heel spurs will lead to chronic swelling and poor surgical outcomes. A better approach is to remove the posterior heel spur in combination with gastrocnemius recession and address the plantar fasciitis with amniotic or platelet-rich plasma injection. Any further invasive plantar fascia surgery could be staged if needed.

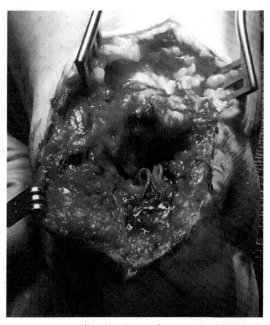

Fig. 1. A difficult-to-manage complication in an obese patient (BMI 45) with a fall rupture of a previously repaired Achilles tendon at the insertion (5 weeks postoperatively).

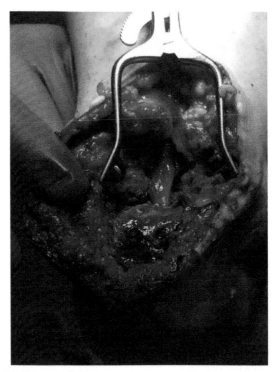

Fig. 2. Revision with FHL transfer.

Perhaps one of the most challenging presentations of foot pain among obese patients is generalized pain throughout the entire foot and ankle. The patient will struggle with isolating the pain to a specific area and will often insist that it hurts all over. These presentations can be very frustrating for the physician because almost no foot and ankle pathologic condition presents this way. Radiographs are useful to rule out fracture or other common pathologic condition. Initial treatment should consist of limited weight-bearing with a walking boot and anti-inflammatory medication. It is hoped that reevaluating the patient after a month will then lead to a more focused complaint that will allow for a definitive diagnosis and treatment plan.

Overall management of foot pain in obese patients is quite challenging. Standards of care are not well established in these situations. Clearly one needs to be open to modifying treatment plans to meet the emerging needs of this patient demographic.

DISCUSSION

Clinical diagnosis of the above discussed types of obesity-related foot pain is mostly observational in nature. Despite difficulties with design study related to obesity and foot pain, various studies on foot pressure and obesity exist. Pirozzi and colleagues[6] showed that as body mass increases, so does foot pressure. One would only expect that as the amount of pressure going through the foot increases so does the chances for this to cause pain. As presented earlier, type 1 and 2 pain mostly involve the midfoot. Walsh and colleagues[7] found that increased body weight leads to increased midfoot pressure. The Walsh study suggested that the midfoot may be the most vulnerable part of the foot for pain when subjected to increased pressure via obesity.

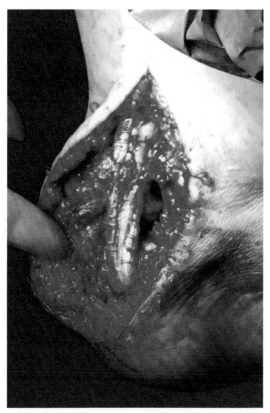

Fig. 3. Revision with FHL transfer and Achilles allograft.

Similarly, Mueller and colleagues[8] showed increased midfoot loading in obese children as compared with nonobese children. Mickle and Steele[9] designed a study to compare pain in patients of normal weight with those who are obese. They found that people with obesity have more foot pain as compared with nonobese patients. They also concluded that obese people have a slower gait, an increased contact time with the ground, and an increased peak pressure across the midfoot.

Obesity and pain have been studied on a molecular level as well. It is thought that excessive adipose tissue leads to increased expression of specific cytokines that perpetuate a chronic state of low-grade inflammation throughout the body. This process is the same process that places a person at risk for hypertension, hypercholesterolemia, and diabetes mellitus.[10,11] Experiments on cartilage show chondrocytes are sensitive to pressure. Chondrocytes respond to increased pressure by expression of cytokines leading to complex biochemical pathways resulting in cartilage destruction and arthritic changes in a joint.[12,13]

A study by Stolzman and colleagues[14] showed increased prevalence of pes planus in children with obesity. Increased body weight contributing to arch collapse intuitively makes sense, and this is seen clinically as discussed earlier in type 3 obesity-related foot pain. Another study showed that weight had more of an effect on causing arch collapse than age.[15] Zhao and colleagues[16] further added to this research by showing foot structure remains unchanged after weight loss. This finding is unfortunate, although reduction in pain can still be expected with weight loss secondary to reducing pressure. Many people function very well and pain free with a flatfoot, so the findings of the Zhao study should not discourage physicians to push for weight loss as a central focus for treating type 3 obesity-related foot pain.

Stavem and colleagues[17] showed that patients with increased BMI are at more of a risk for developing Weber type C ankle fractures. These fractures are traditionally unstable, and in combination with increased body weight, this can make it quite difficult to properly treat these patients. Furthermore, Shibuya and colleagues[18] published on obesity as being a risk factor for open ankle fractures. Obesity is a well-documented risk factor for developing deep venous thrombosis.[19] Total ankle implant surgery is also complicated by obesity as a 17.8% revision rate has been reported.[20]

Compliance with postoperative non-weight-bearing protocols can be a challenge for obese patients. These patients are clearly at risk for falling, which could affect the surgical site or lead to a new injury. Preoperative evaluation by a physical therapist is ideal and has been shown to be helpful for other orthopedic-related procedures involving the hip and knee.[21] It is best for the patient to have all needed durable medical equipment before surgery and to already know how to use it. In addition, lymphedema should be considered for evaluation through referral to a lymphedema clinic before surgery. These clinics can help reduce the level of swelling to the lower extremities, which will make casting the patient much easier.

The authors recommend that foot and ankle surgeons test all patients for vitamin D deficiency before foot and ankle surgery. From the bariatric literature, it has been shown that 90% of patients undergoing weight loss surgery are vitamin D deficient.[22] This topic has been researched thoroughly because it was thought that this issue would be even worse following gastric bypass surgery secondary to malabsorption. However, bariatric research has shown that following weight loss surgery there is significant improvement in vitamins D levels. These findings suggest that increased weight alone may be a cause of vitamin D deficiency.[23] **Fig. 4** shows subtalar joint nonunion in a patient with a BMI of 35 and vitamin D deficiency with type 1 obesity-related foot pain.

Seeing as how this group of patients is at a higher risk for the development of postoperative complications, vigilance is essential in regards to preoperative evaluation and consultation (see **Fig. 4**). Standard blood work should be obtained, including a complete blood count, basic metabolic panel, and vitamin D level. Medical evaluation and optimization from the patient's primary care physician should be obtained as well as any other needed consultations or specialty testing, such as cardiology and cardiac stress testing, respectively. Preoperative evaluation by the physical therapist, as discussed earlier, is essential to avoid procedure failure and to expedite and facilitate a patient's recovery. Smoking cessation at least 1 month before surgery is necessary, and nicotine levels should be checked to confirm. If at any point during this preoperative phase the patient seems unwilling to comply with any portion of the preoperative workup, then surgery should be delayed or avoided all together. The inability of a patient to comply with these basic preoperative requirements oftentimes will lead the surgeon down the correct path of not performing the surgery.

This discussion would be incomplete without addressing the topic of diet. It is beneficial to discuss weight loss with patients before any planned elective procedures.[24] Recommendation of a specific diet is somewhat controversial and complicated. It is not the goal of this article to thoroughly address this but rather give the reader a different perspective. In general, very little time is spent in medical school educating students on diet and nutrition. Academically there is a paucity of education on this topic, and in many instances, physicians are the biggest culprits when it comes to

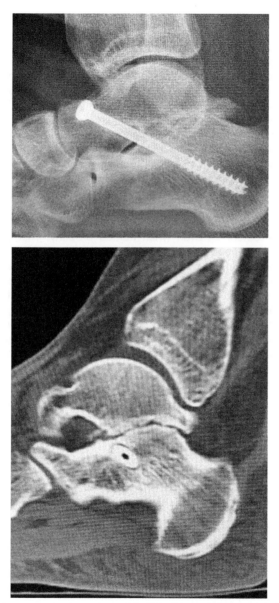

Fig. 4. Subtalar joint nonunion in patient with BMI of 35 and vitamin D deficiency, with type 1 obesity-related foot pain.

an unhealthy diet, very much like the smoking physician who lectures a patient to stop smoking. In addition, many foot and ankle surgeons assume that primary care physicians are educating patients on appropriate diet, but unfortunately this is not always the case. Most patients have been told to eat less and exercise more. This approach gives very little guidance. Not only are patients unable to exercise due to foot pain, but the ability to "eat less" or "everything in moderation" proves to be difficult and unsustainable, and clearly is not effective. Initially opening up a conversation with these patients can be challenging, and the physician should proceed with some caution. It is not uncommon for people to become emotional when any discussion on weight is brought up, although these patients usually seem very appreciative that you actually took time to talk to them about this as other physicians have avoided it altogether. Patients who seem uninterested in discussing diet are usually not going to get much out of any discussion on diet. The senior author recommends a whole foods plant-based diet to patients and is prepared to discuss this with them at length. This plant-based approach is safe and allows a sustainable diet that is naturally a low-calorie diet, allowing patients to avoid the hassle of calorie counting.

Obesity presents a significant challenge to the foot and ankle surgeon. In many instances, avoiding surgery is the best approach even if this upsets this group of patients. In cases where surgery is to be performed, oftentimes the surgeon is obligated to adjust the standard surgical approach by adding additional procedures or performing a different type of procedure, that is, fusion instead of periarticular osteotomy. Obese patients are at risk for postoperative complications and often have bad surgical outcomes even when treated properly. This additional risk in regards to a higher complication rate, increased severity, and advanced difficulty in revision experienced in the obese patient population should be discussed with the patient preoperatively. Open communication with the patient serves as a way to educate the patient and potentially influence a given patient to attempt reduction of increased complications via weight loss. This weight loss may, in fact, obviate surgery. Physicians need to place more importance on understanding nutrition so they can have more meaningful discussion with patients in regard to their diets, weight loss, and lifestyle modifications. Unfortunately, obesity seems to be a problem that is only getting worse. This issue is guaranteed to continue to challenge the foot and ankle physician for years to come.

REFERENCES

1. Available at: www.who.int. Accessed July 1, 2018.
2. Available at: www.cdc.gov/obesity/. Accessed July 1, 2018.
3. Wang Y, Beydoun MA, Laing L, et al. Will all Americans become overweight or obese? Estimating the progression and cost of the US obesity epidemic. Obesity (Silver Spring) 2008;16(10):2323–30.
4. Butterworth PA, Landorf KB, Gilleard W, et al. The association between body composition and foot structure and function: a systemic review. Obes Rev 2014;15(4):348–57.
5. Ficke B, Elattar O, Naranje SM, et al. Gastrocnemius recession for recalcitrant plantar fasciitis in overweight and obese patients. Foot Ankle Surg 2017 [pii:S1268-7731(17)30111-X].
6. Pirozzi K, McGuire J, Meyer A. Effect of variable bonds mass on plantar foot pressure and off-loading device efficacy. J Foot Ankle Surg 2014;14:588–97.
7. Walsh TP, Butterworth PA, Urquhart DM, et al. Increase in body weight over a 2 year period is associated with an increase in midfoot pressure and foot pain. J Foot Ankle Res 2017;10:21.
8. Mueller S, Carlsohn A, Mueller J, et al. Influence of obesity on foot loading characteristics in gait for children 1-12 years. PLoS One 2016;11(2):e0149924.
9. Mickle KJ, Steele JR. Obese older adults suffer foot pain and foot related functional limitation. Gait Posture 2015;42(4):442–7.

10. Katz JD, Agrawal S, Velasquez M. Getting to the heart of the matter: osteoarthritis takes its place as part of the metabolic syndrome. Curr Opin Rheumatol 2010; 22(5):512–9.
11. Yoshimura N, Muraki S, Oka H, et al. Association of knees osteoarthritis with the accumlation of metabolic risk factors such as overweight, hypertension, dyslipidemia, and impaired glucose tolerance in Japanese men and women: the ROAD stud. J Rheumatol 2011;38(5):921–30.
12. Pottie P, Presle N, Terlain B, et al. Obesity and osteoarthritis: more complex than predicted. Ann Rheum Dis 2006;65(11):1404–5.
13. Guilak F, Fermor B, Keene FJ, et al. The role of biomechanics and inflammation in cartilage injury and repair. Clin Orthop Relat Res 2004;423:17–26.
14. Stolzman S, Irby MB, Callahan AB, et al. Pes planus and paediatric obesity: a Systematic review. Clin Obes 2015;5(2):52–9.
15. Jankowicz-Szymanska A, Wodka K, Kolpa M, et al. Foot longitudinal arches in obese, overweight and normal weight females who differ in age. Homo 2018; 69(1–2):37–42.
16. Zhao X, Tsujimoto T, Kim B, et al. Increasing physical activity might be more effective to improve foot structure and function than weight reduction in obese adults. J Foot Ankle Surg 2018;57(5):876–9.
17. Stavem K, Neumann M, Sigurdsen U. Association of body mass index with the pattern of surgically treated ankle fractures using two classification systems. J Foot Ankle Surg 2016;56(2):314–8.
18. Shibuya N, Liu G, Davis M. Risk factor of open malleolar fractures: an analysis of the national trauma data bank (2007-2011). J Foot Ankle Surg 2015;55(1):94–8.
19. Fleischer A, Abicht B, Baker J. American college of foot and ankle surgeons clinical consensus statement: risk, prevention, and diagnosis of venous thromboembolism disease in foot and ankle surgery and injuries requiring immobilization. J Foot Ankle Surg 2015;54(3):497–507.
20. Sansosti LE, Van J, Meyr A. Effect of obesity on total ankle arthroplasty: a systematic review of postoperative complication requiring surgical revision. J Foot Ankle Surg 2017;57(2):353–6.
21. Snow R, Granata J, Ruhil AV, et al. Association between preoperative physical therapy and post acute care utilization patterns and cost in total joint replacement. J Bone Joint Surg Am 2014;96(19):e165.
22. Goldberg WS, Stoner JA, Thompson J, et al. Prevalence of vitamin D insufficiency and deficiency in morbidly obese patients: a comparison with non obese controls. Obese Surg 2008;18(2):145–50.
23. Coupaye M, Breuil MC, Riviere P, et al. Serum vitamin D increases with weight loss in obese subjects 6 months after Roux-en-Y gastric bypass. Obese Surg 2013;23(4):486–93.
24. Stewart M. Obesity in elective foot and ankle surgery. Orthop Clin North Am 2018; 49:371–9.

Postoperative Convalescence

Doug Richie, DPM[a,b,c,*], Daniel Bullard, DPM[d]

KEYWORDS

- Postoperative convalescence • Gait training • Non–weight bearing • Mobility
- Durable medical equipment • Hygiene • Nutrition • Sleep aides

KEY POINTS

- Preparation for the postoperative period preoperatively may help to avoid adversity along course of recovery.
- Appropriate communication between the physician and the patient in terms of disability the patient may expect postoperatively will assist in the limitation and potentially avoidance of postoperative convalescence problems related to activities of daily living.
- It is important to be explicit in terms of length and type of disability imposed by the postoperative requirements of a specific surgery.
- Preoperative communication and planning are essential to be prepared to address issues surrounding nutrition, hygiene, mobility, and sleeping during the postoperative course.
- It is important to identify and obtain appropriate durable medical equipment for successful and safe performance of activities of daily living after surgery.

INTRODUCTION

Planning for a patient's needs with regard to postoperative convalescence helps assure a successful surgical outcome. When the podiatric surgeon considers the suitability of a patient to undergo surgery, the decision making is often focused only on medical risk factors. The preoperative consultation should cover a multitude of surgical parameters, such as discussion of risk-to-benefit ratio of a particular procedure, the exact nature of that procedure, anesthesia involved for the completion of the

Disclosure Statements: The authors have nothing to disclose.
[a] Private Practice, Alamitos-Seal Beach Podiatry Group, 550 Pacific Coast Highway, Suite 209, Seal Beach, CA 90740, USA; [b] Department of Biomechanics, California School of Podiatric Medicine at Samuel Merritt University, Oakland, CA, USA; [c] Western University of Health Sciences, Pomona, CA, USA; [d] St Vincent Charity Medical Center, 2322 East 22nd Street, Cleveland, OH 44115, USA
* Corresponding author. 550 Pacific Coast Highway, Suite 209, Seal Beach, CA 90740.
E-mail address: drichiejr@aol.com

procedure, and patient requirements needed for successful healing of the procedure. However, proportionally, most of the discussion between the physician and the patient is centered on the indications and the technical nature involved with a given surgery. If a thorough interview is not conducted with the patient to determine their capability in complying with all of the restrictions placed after surgery, the outcome could be compromised or end in failure. This specifically applies to a patient's ability to perform activities of daily living, such as bathing, using the restroom, and eating, while attempting to comply with necessary gait and activity restrictions to allow for adequate healing of proposed musculoskeletal surgery.

The discussion should begin with a detailed description of the disability imposed by the particular surgery and the length of time the disability will be in place. Besides simply stating that "you will not be able to bear weight your foot for 6 weeks," it is critical to outline what this restriction will do to the patient's activities of daily living. "Because you are going to be non–weight bearing, how are you going to prepare meals? How are you going to bathe or shower? How are you going to get in and out of your car? If we operate on your right foot, you must realize that you cannot drive for 4 to 6 weeks."

Many disciplines have noted the beneficial effects of preoperative assessment, education, and prehabilitation to address a variety of patient-driven prerequisites necessary for successful procedure completion. One of the most notable is the process of "joint camp" for patients experiencing total joint replacement surgery of the knee or hip. Although there is no significant need for "joint camp" as a general rule with regard to foot and ankle surgery, the same approach should be undertaken with respect to evaluating, educating, and preemptively training the patient regarding all aspects of a particular foot and ankle surgery. This process should be included on any practitioner's preoperative work sheet and become part of a standard surgical consultation. By doing this, all parties involved, staff, surgeon, and patient, will be engaged in this prehabilitation process, which will increase chances of success.

It is appropriate to inquire about the availability of family, friends, or other people to act as caregivers during the recovery period. If there is no help available, consideration should be made to cancel or postpone the surgery. In some cases, educating the patient about durable medical equipment (DME) options and home health aides could make the difference between canceling or perhaps moving forward. Furthermore, use of these devices can many times make the difference between a surgical failure and a successful outcome. If a patient gives up on keeping the extremity non–weight bearing or falls in the shower, a perfect surgical procedure will suddenly become a complication or failed procedure.

The postoperative activities of daily living focus on 4 areas: mobility, nutrition, sleeping, and hygiene. All are essential for well-being and all are negatively impacted by many foot and ankle surgical procedures. Here is a list of options that can make the postoperative period far safer and more manageable for any patient undergoing foot and ankle surgery (Appendices 1–3). These options can solve many of the challenges that affect mobility, nutrition, and hygiene during the postoperative recovery.

MOBILITY
Coping with a Non–weight-Bearing Status

Many foot and ankle surgeries require avoidance of weight bearing on the affected extremity for an extended period. This can be a daunting task for all but the few young and athletic patients who undergo elective foot and ankle surgery. Because most foot and ankle surgical patients are older than 30, maintaining a total non–weight-bearing status on a lower extremity can be almost impossible. This may explain the nonunion rates seen with midfoot, hindfoot, and ankle fusion procedures. These patients promise to follow guidelines, but lack the physical ability to be compliant in this regard. Some options, with pros and cons, for ambulating while keeping one lower extremity non–weight bearing are as follows:

Crutches

Pro: Maneuverable in tight spaces in the home setting. Easy to store.
Con: Requires good upper body strength and coordination.
   Hazardous on wet surfaces.
Consider: Ergonomic crutches, which relieve some stress on the arms.

iWalk

Pro: Eliminates need for upper body strength.
   Frees up the hands for kitchen, hygiene, and so forth.
   Can climb and descend stairs.
   Can reduce energy drain seen with crutches.
Con: Requires balance and dexterity.
Consider: Refer the patient to a local DME facility for fitting and a test trial with the iWalk before surgery.

Knee-scooter

Pro: Minimal need for strength, coordination.
   Minimal depletion of energy.
Con: Are unstable and can be a fall hazard.
   Can aggravate knee conditions.
   Bulky, may be challenging to store in car.
   Difficult to navigate in the home setting.
Consider: Using a knee-scooter only when long periods of ambulation are needed.

Implementing Protective Offloading Devices

Whether a full, partial, or non–weight-bearing postoperative protocol is implemented, most patients are required to wear a protective device on the operated extremity. Postoperative surgical shoes and walking boots are most popular and fall under a category of DME often dispensed by the operating physician. Surgical shoes are billed under code L3260. Surgical shoes have limited ability to offload the metatarsals. Pressure studies have shown that surgical shoes can reduce peak plantar pressures under the metatarsals by 30%, whereas standard shoes will reduce these pressures by only 10%.[1,2]

Walking boots offload plantar pressures at the forefoot by up to 80%,[3] but not all walking boots offer the same mechanical effects. Immobilizing devices are used to reduce stress across surgical sites. Reducing plantar pressure or loads across the bones and soft tissues of the feet is one purpose of offloading devices. Reducing motion across the ankle, hindfoot, and forefoot joints is another purpose. Kadakia and colleagues[4] studied various forms of offloading to determine effects on ankle joint motion. A fiberglass cast will allow 8° of sagittal plane motion across the ankle joint. A pneumatic walking boot with anterior shell will allow 15° of ankle joint motion, and a nonpneumatic boot will allow 19° of motion. A low-top (half-leg) walking boot allows 39° of motion.[4]

Besides the mechanical differences, there are different billing codes for walking boots. Pneumatic walking boots are billed using code L4361, whereas nonpneumatic walking boots are billed using code L4387. These codes are recommended as most relevant to the podiatric practice, as the fitting of walking boots requires minimal adjustment.

There are challenges when billing for walking boots for the surgical patient. For a trauma patient, a walking boot will usually be dispensed before surgery, and the medical necessity for the device has already been established. However, for the elective surgical patient undergoing a procedure such as a Lapidus bunionectomy, the medical necessity for the walking boot is not established until after the surgical procedure has been performed. Medicare and many private insurers will not cover the walking boot until the medical necessity has been established. It is preferable to dispense crutches and walking boots to the elective foot and ankle surgery patient before the surgery. This is particularly helpful in crutch training and proper education for fitting and adjustment of the walking boot on the presurgical office visit. However, it would not be appropriate to bill a third-party payer on that day for the DME devices. One solution would be to collect a deposit from the patient to cover the cost of the devices, and then wait until the surgical day to submit the billing to the carrier.

Another concern with walking boots, casts, and even surgical shoes is the potential to compromise balance during standing and walking. Numerous studies have shown this potential effect, particularly with patients who are already compromised by age or neuropathy. Shoes with rocker bottom soles, a common feature in postsurgical shoes, have been shown to compromise balance and postural control.[5] Walking boots will significantly affect balance in older patients and patients with neuropathy.[6–8] An effective offset to the negative effects on balance posed by casts and walking boots is the use of a cane. A cane improves balance and steadiness in gait for several reasons. Studies have shown that the upper extremity can provide proprioceptive input to improve postural control when the lower extremities are impaired by peripheral neuropathy.[9,10] When patients are given a cane, stability in gait improves.[11] This improvement might also be a simple mechanical effect, as patients can bear up to 25% of body weight on a cane during unipedal stance and undergoing perturbation.[12]

There are other assistive devices that can be used to improve stability in gait and provide partial offloading of the operated extremity. Consider a walker or a rollator. A rollator is essentially a walker with wheels. Many models have a seat that allows the rollator to be converted to a transport chair.

NUTRITION

Upright standing is often prohibited in the immediate postsurgical foot and ankle patient. Thus, meal preparation can be challenging. A rollator can be an option for the patient to remain seated while preparing meals. A knee-scooter is another option, but requires more balance than a rollator. Patients should be cautioned about their limitations in the kitchen during the postoperative recovery. This can allow the patient opportunity to plan ahead with advance meal preparation. Before surgery, preparing a week's worth of meals that can be prepared ahead of time or stocking quick microwave-ready meals can solve a lot of challenges.

At the same time, adequate intake of proper nutrition must be emphasized to ensure optimal healing from the surgical procedure. Patients must be encouraged to eat well-balanced meals 3 times daily, even if this poses a physical challenge involved with the preparation of meals. Preoperatively, this is an issue in which it is essential to arrange for assistance from family members or neighbors to avoid compromising situations in the kitchen while preparing meals. It is not uncommon for this aspect of postoperative recovery to be neglected until after the surgery. Although the appetite is depressed in the immediate postoperative period (24 hours) in many cases due to anesthetic agents and/or pain medications, resumption of regular eating habits is essential not only for surgical healing but also for maintenance of baseline health, as many of these patients are medically compromised and cannot tolerate prolonged periods without appropriate nutrition. In some cases, hiring a caregiver in the home will be necessary to ensure that the patient is fed and avoids compromising situations in the kitchen. Another option is to investigate whether meals on wheels is available for a given patient.

SLEEPING

Getting in and out of bed can be a daunting task when a patient is immobilized in a boot or cast, and when the patient is in significant pain. Often, patients prefer to stay in bed and avoid getting up to eat, bathe, and use the bathroom. There are options to assist them with this task.

There are a variety of bedrails available for rent from DME stores that can be affixed to an existing bed and provide an effective aid for getting in and out of bed. There are bedrails with an adjustable cane or pole to allow grasping, and these devices are particularly useful when transferring to a wheelchair. A bedrail option is available that has a tray for eating or working on a computer. For more debilitating surgery, it may be necessary to rent a trapeze bar, which can be installed on some beds. In other cases, renting a true hospital bed with trapeze may be necessary.

Elevation of the operated extremity is often recommended after foot and ankle surgery. Rather than using unstable pillows, a bed wedge can be purchased or rented, which is effective and safer than a stack of pillows.

Surgical patients should consider the challenge of getting dressed while immobilized in a boot or cast and potentially maintaining non–weight-bearing status on the affected extremity. Furthermore, postsurgical pain may limit ability to bend over, grasp clothing, or pull clothing over an operated extremity. Devices that may ease these tasks include buttoning aids, zipper pulls, shoe horns with long handle, sock aids, dressing sticks, and reachers. This is also an area in which family members will be invaluable to assist with an important task to expedite as well as to perform as safely as possible.

HYGIENE

Almost all surgical procedures require keeping the operative site clean and dry for 7 to 14 days. At the same time, hygiene requires daily bathing. The preoperative patient should be asked to evaluate his or her options to fulfill these needs while compromised with postoperative restrictions.

How often will patients tell you how difficult it is to get up from the toilet when they are to be non–weight bearing and wearing a walking boot? What are some solutions? One option is to rent suction-tipped grab bars that can be placed around the toilet. Toilet seat risers can reduce the demand for bending. In some cases, the patient will be better off with a bedside commode with grab bars.

Bathing is a more daunting challenge for the postsurgical patient, particularly when required to be non–weight bearing. Keeping the dressings dry can now be accomplished with use of commercial cast-protector bags, which are easy to use and are very effective.

Stepping in and out of the shower can be aided by use of pivoting shower benches or chairs. Grab bars are highly recommended, but many patients have not already have them in their showers and are reluctant to install them. Suction tip grab bars are available to place in and outside the shower. A better option is to recommend tub baths in which a grab bar can be slipped over the side of the tub and swivel or pivoting bath chairs are easier to use than in the shower. A transfer bench or board is easy to place across the bathtub and can provide seating and a stable surface to slide across when entering and exiting the bath. Most bath and shower seats are height adjustable and can be used in the kitchen for seating during meal preparation. In short, adjustable bath or shower seats are highly recommended for all podiatric surgical patients.

PREOPERATIVE PHYSICAL THERAPY

Therapy in the preoperative setting focuses on assessing functionality and potential limitations during the postoperative course. Theoretically, any potential limitation, if identified early, can be addressed with strength training, gait training, and appropriate DME selection. The literature regarding preoperative physical therapy for foot and ankle surgery is sparse; however, it does indicate that substantial improvements in strength and functionality can be gained before the postoperative period. However, this does not consistently demonstrate improvements in functional recovery. A vast majority of this literature stems from articles focusing on total hip/knee replacements.

There have been multiple attempts to assess preoperative strength training for patients undergoing total hip and total knee replacements, including a systematic review; however, the only gains in functionality are with regard to length of hospital stay. In fact, the only available systematic review on preoperative training demonstrates that there is no difference in functional recovery in patients undergoing total knee replacements despite significant improvements in strength.[13] However, initiating physical therapy on postoperative day 1 does result in reduced hospital stays, which can potentially improve outcomes by avoiding hospital-based complications.[14]

Even individualized home-based physical therapy fails to demonstrate functional improvement in patients undergoing total knee arthroplasty. In a study by Oosting and colleagues,[15] patients underwent 3 to 6 weeks of individual home-based therapy twice a week for 30 minutes versus group physical therapy at a local hospital 3 times a week. Personalized, home-based therapy provides advantages with regard to progressive escalation of training, better functional monitoring, and adaptation to the patient's unique living situation. Both groups included education regarding the operation, functional assessments, and crutch training. When assessing the patient preoperatively, but at the completion of therapy, statistically significant improvements in 6-minute walk test, chair-rise test, patient-specific complaints, and pain levels were shown in the home-based physical therapy group when compared with usual preoperative training protocols.[15] At 2 to 4 days after hospital discharge, no difference between groups with regard to functional recovery was demonstrated, and at 6 weeks after discharge both groups demonstrated diffuse functional improvements relative to their prior assessment.[15] Patients who underwent the home-based individualized therapies failed to outperform the usual preoperative physical therapy protocol in all functional categories except for chair-rise time.[15]

Despite the lack of evidence for preoperative physical therapy providing improved functional recovery, literature has shown that preoperative gait training may address any mechanical defects, which can arguably result in better postoperative outcomes. In a study, 5 patients with significant knee hyperextension issues throughout the stance period were encouraged to focus on walking with their knees flexed, maintaining ankle joint dorsiflexion, and maintaining an erect posture. This resulted in a 79% reduction in knee extension (stance), 30% reduction in medial tibiofemoral loads, and a significant reduction in adduction/abduction moments about the knee and ankle joint plantarflexion.[13] Preoperative gait training is an opportunity to address biomechanical faults in an attempt to promote improved long-term outcomes.

REFERENCES

1. Fleischli JG, Lavery LA, Vela SA, et al. 1997 William J. Stickel Bronze Award. Comparison of strategies for reducing pressure at the site of neuropathic ulcers. J Am Podiatr Med Assoc 1997;87:466.
2. Lavery LA, Vela SA, Lavery DC, et al. Reducing dynamic foot pressures in high-risk diabetics with foot ulcerations: a comparison of treatments. Diabetes Care 1996;19:818–21.
3. Cavanagh PR, Bus SA. Off-loading the diabetic foot for ulcer prevention and healing. J Am Podiatr Med Assoc 2010;100(5):360–8.
4. Kadakia AR, Espinosa N, Smerek J, et al. Radiographic comparison of sagittal plane stability between cast and boots. Foot Ankle Int 2008;29:421–6.
5. Albright BC, Woodhul-Smith WM. Rocker bottom soles alter the postural response to backward translation during stance. Gait Posture 2009;30:45–9.
6. Bennell K, Coldie A. The differential effects of external ankle support on postural control. J Orthop Sports Phys Ther 1994;20:287–95.
7. Lavery LA, Fleishli JG, Laughlin TJ, et al. Is postural instability exacerbated by off-loading devices in high risk diabetics with foot ulcers? Ostomy Wound Manage 1998;44:26–32, 34.
8. Hijmans JM, Geertzen JHB, Dijkstra PU, et al. A systematic review of the effects of shoes and other ankle or foot appliances on balance in older people and people with peripheral nervous system disorders. Gait Posture 2007;25: 316–23.
9. Jeka JJ. Light touch as a balance aid. Phys Ther 1997;77:476–87.
10. Dickstein R, Shupert CL, Horak FB. Fingertip touch improves postural stability in patients with peripheral neuropathy. Gait Posture 2001;14:238–47.
11. Sainsbury R, Mulley GP. Walking sticks used by the elderly. BMJ 1982;284:1751.
12. Ashton-Miller JA, Yeh MWL, Richardson JK, et al. A cane reduces loss of balance in patients with peripheral neuropathy: results from a challenging unipedal balance test. Arch Phys Med Rehabil 1996;77:446–52.
13. Ma J-X, Zhang L-K, Kuang M-J, et al. The effect of preoperative training on functional recovery in patients undergoing total knee arthroplasty: a systematic review and meta-analysis. Int J Surg 2018;51:205–12.
14. Juliano K, Edwards D, Spinello D, et al. Initiating physical therapy on the day of surgery decreases length of stay without compromising functional outcomes following total hip arthroplasty. HSS J 2010;7(1):16–20.
15. Oosting E, Jans MP, Dronkers JJ, et al. Preoperative home-based physical therapy versus usual care to improve functional health of frail older adults scheduled for elective total hip arthroplasty: a pilot randomized controlled trial. Arch Phys Med Rehabil 2012;93(4):610–6.

APPENDIX 1: AMBULATORY AIDS: PATIENT EQUIPMENT LIST: FOOT AND ANKLE SURGERY

Crutches
  Ergonomic handle crutches
  Plush saddle crutches
  Standard

Crutch Alternatives
  iWalk
  Knee scooters

Walkers
  3-Wheel
  4-Wheel
  Push Walkers
  In-Step rollators

Wheelchair
  Transporter
  Wheelchair with footrest

Cane
  Standard
  4-prong
  Cane seat

APPENDIX 2: BEDROOM: PATIENT EQUIPMENT LIST: FOOT AND ANKLE SURGERY

Dressing Aids
  Buttoning aids
  Zipper pulls
  Shoe horns: long handle
  Dressing sticks
  Reachers
  Shoelaces: coiled and elastic

Bed
  Bedrails
  Bedrails with built-in cane
  Bedrails with magazine holder
  Patient lift
  Trapeze bar
  Handrails
  Over-the-bed swivel trays
  Leg wedges
  Bed wedges

APPENDIX 3: BATHROOM: PATIENT EQUIPMENT LIST: FOOT AND ANKLE SURGERY

Dressing and Cast Care
  Shower protector

Seating
  Bath/Shower chairs
  Transfer benches
  Sliding transfer benches

Pivoting benches
Bath lifts
Folding shower seats
Bath mats

Toilet
Toilet seat risers
Toilet safety rails
Bidets
Commodes: wheeled, drop-arm, heavy duty

Grab Bars
Standard grab bars
Suction grip grab bars
Bathtub grab bars

Printed and bound by CPI Group (UK) Ltd, Croydon, CR0 4YY

03/10/2024

01040394-0012